SpringerBriefs in Cancer Research

For further volumes:
http://www.springer.com/series/10786

Natalia Aptsiauri • Angel Miguel Garcia-Lora
Teresa Cabrera

MHC Class I Antigens In Malignant Cells

Immune Escape and Response to Immunotherapy

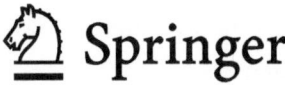 Springer

Natalia Aptsiauri
Servicio de Análisis Clínicos
Hosp. Universitario Virgen de las Nieves
Granada, Spain

Angel Miguel Garcia-Lora
Servicio de Análisis Clínicos
Hosp. Universitario Virgen de las Nieves
Granada, Spain

Teresa Cabrera
Departamento de Bioquímica y Biología
    Molecular III e Inmunología
Universidad de Granada
Granada, Spain

ISBN 978-1-4614-6542-3   ISBN 978-1-4614-6543-0 (eBook)
DOI 10.1007/978-1-4614-6543-0
Springer New York Heidelberg Dordrecht London

Library of Congress Control Number: 2013931654

Springer is part of Springer Science+Business Media (www.springer.com)

Acknowledgments

We would like to thank David Diez Cabrera a professional artist for the figures. We would also like to acknowledge all the contributions of the students and investigators who have been part of the large research group at the Department of Clinical Analysis at the Virgen de las Nieves University Hospital in Granada, Spain. This work has been supported over the years by grants from the Fondo de Investigaciones Sanitarias (FIS), Red Genomica del Cancer (RETIC), Plan Andaluz de Investigación (Group CTS-143), Servicio Andaluz de Salud (SAS), Plan Nacional de Investigación Científica, Desarrollo e Innovación Tecnológica (Proyectos SAF 2007-63262, and SAF 2010-20273) in Spain; and from different European projects.

Acknowledgments

Contents

Chapter 1
Overview of MHC Class I Antigens

Cancer development is the result of an accumulation of genetic alterations. Activation or inactivation of certain genes (proto-oncogenes and tumor suppressor genes) is required for cell transformation. As a result of these genetic alterations, tumor cells produce new or modified proteins that are processed by the cell, generating small peptides that enter the route of Major Histocompatibility Complex (MHC) class I for presentation to T cells. Cytotoxic and helper T lymphocytes recognize antigenic peptides processed and presented by MHC class I and II molecules, respectively. Therefore, T cells have the ability to monitor any genetic alteration, including those associated with malignant transformation.

MHC Class I Genes and Molecules

MHC class I molecules are cell surface glycoproteins composed of two non-covalently associated polypeptide subunits (Cresswel et al. 1973), a polymorphic chain of 45 kDa (heavy chain or α chain) and a non-polymorphic protein 12 kDa, called β2-microglobulin (β2m). The antigenic peptide is assembled with this structure, resulting in a peptide-MHC class I complex. Extracellular region of the heavy chain is divided into three domains: α1, α2, and α3. The peptide binding groove is formed as an interchain dimer by folding of α1 and α2 domains to create a long cleft, where polymorphic amino acid residues cluster in hypervariable regions (Stern and Wiley 1994). Thus, the groove formed by these domains anchor the peptide recognized by the T cell receptor (TCR).

MHC molecules in human are called Human Leucocyte Antigens (HLA). The genes encoding heavy chain are located on the short arm of chromosome 6 in humans and in chromosome 17 in mouse. The β2m gene is independent from MHC (or HLA) complex and is located on chromosome 15 in human and chromosome 2 in mouse (Goodfellow et al. 1975).

N. Aptsiauri et al., *MHC Class I Antigens In Malignant Cells: Immune Escape and Response to Immunotherapy*, SpringerBriefs in Cancer Research 6, DOI 10.1007/978-1-4614-6543-0_1, © Teresa Cabrera 2013

The HLA system is a genetic region that is divided into different sub-regions or closely linked loci. They are inherited in a Mendelian co-dominant form giving rise to the most polymorphic antigenic system that exists in humans. Within the class I region three genes called classical (HLA-A,-B,-C), and three non-classic (HLA-E, -F,-G) (Geraghty 1993) are distinguished. Therefore, each person expresses a combination of six HLA class I classic alleles on majority of their cells. However, when we look at the population in general, hundreds of alleles for each locus can be found (Robinson et al. 2011).

MHC genes in the mouse are known as H-2 genes. Due to the small size of the H-2 complex genetic recombination is rare, and each pair of alleles is transferred from one generation to another as a set. The alleles transferred together as a unit in each chromosome are called a haplotype. The haplotypes of the most commonly used strains are standard and have assigned certain alleles. For example, BALB/c strain has H-2^d haplotype, whereas C57/BL6 mice have H-2^b haplotype. There are three H-2 class-I molecules: K, D, and L, and are located in K and D regions of the complex. They correspond to HLA-A, B, and C molecules in the human HLA complex and also consist of a heavy α chain and β2-microglobulin. The molecules K and D are expressed in all haplotypes, but the number of L loci expressed in the different haplotypes range from none (H-2^b) to three (H-2^k).

MHC Class I Antigen Processing, Transport, and Assembly

Antigen presentation on the plasma membrane is only the last step of a chain of events known as antigen processing occurring within the cell, where the MHC molecules are involved in active form. MHC class I molecules are involved mainly in endogenous antigen processing, such as the products of viral components in virus-infected cells (Townsend and Bodmer 1989). On the contrary, class II molecules act mostly during the processing of exogenous antigens, previously captured by the cell via endocytosis (Chicz et al. 1992). In any case, the first event to consider is the proteolytic degradation of the antigens into small fragments, capable of forming stable complexes with corresponding MHC molecules. Antigens, which are originally found in the cytosol, are degraded by proteolytic enzymes into short length fragments (8–10 amino-acid residues) (Rotzschke et al. 1990; Falk et al. 1991). In this enzymatic fragmentation the complex known as proteasome plays an important role. The proteasome consists of a cylindrical 20S proteolytic core complex capped at one or both ends by 19S regulatory complexes, that deubiquitinates and unfolds substrates before translocating them into its core for proteolysis (Amerik and Hochstrasser 2004; Pickart and Cohen 2004). Next, peptides are transported into endoplasmic reticulum (ER) by action of TAP-1 and TAP-2 transporters (Monaco 1992; Shepherd et al. 1993) (see Fig. 1.1).

During the immune response, interferon-γ producing cells (activated T lymphocytes and NK cells) along with an increase in transcription of MHC and TAP genes induce production of three ß catalytic subunits: LMP2 (ß1i), LMP7 (ß5i), and

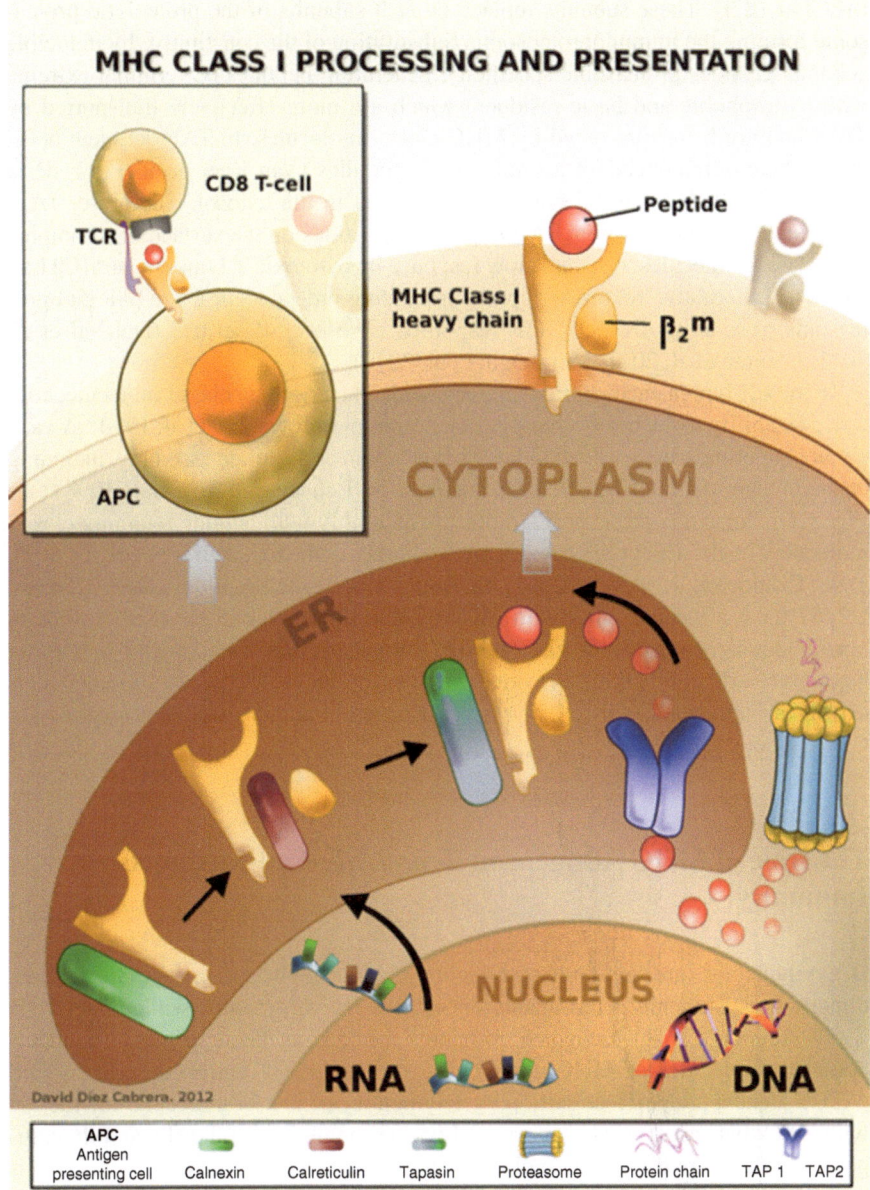

Fig. 1.1 MHC class I intracellular assembly and transport to the cell surface. Ubiquitinated proteins are degraded by the proteasome (or immunoproteasome) into peptides. These peptides are translocated into the ER by the transporter associated with antigen processing, which consists of two subunits, TAP1 and TAP2. In the ER peptides are further trimmed by ER aminopeptidase and bind to HLA class I/β2m complex with the help of chaperone tapasin. The HLA class I/β2m complex formation in the ER is carried out with the help of chaperones: ERp57, calnexin, and calreticulin. The stable HLA class I/β2m complex is subsequently transported via the Golgi system to the cell surface, where peptides are presented for recognition by the cytotoxic CD8+ T-cells via T-cell receptor (TCR)

MECL-1 (ß2i). These subunits replace other ß subunits of the proteolytic protea-some forming the immunoproteosome. Substitution of the constitutive by inducible subunits changes proteasome specificity, generating peptides (C-terminal extreme with hydrophobic and basic residues) which are more effectively transported by TAPs and are better presented by MHC class I molecules. In TAP-deficient cells, class I heterodimers cannot assemble with peptides (Van Kaer et al. 1992; de la Salle et al. 1994), being unstable and degraded in the cytosol. Therefore, TAP-deficient cells do not present TAP-dependent peptides on the surface in a complex with class I molecules, causing a low response by cytotoxic T lymphocytes (CTLs). However, alternative routes of peptide processing independent from TAP and pro-teasome generating distinct CTLs responses have been described (Del Val et al. 2011; Lorente et al. 2011; Merzougui et al. 2011).

In the ER lumen each peptide interacts with a heavy chain class I molecule, con-ferring stability to the heavy chain-β2m heterodimer (Townsend et al. 1990). A vari-ety of chaperones are involved in heavy chain-β2m and peptide assembly, including calnexin, calreticulin, ERp57/ER60, and tapasin (Lehner and Trowsdale 1998) (see Fig. 1.1). Tapasin controls MHC molecule assembly with peptide retaining class I molecules in the ER until they acquire peptides with high affinity (Lehner et al. 1998; Grandea and Van Kaer 2001). In the absence of such peptides calreticulin and ERp57 have a weaker bond with class I heterodimers (Grandea et al. 2000). In tapasin-deficient mice most class I MHC molecules are loaded with low affinity peptides (Garbi et al. 2000). Provided with appropriate stability, class I molecule is driven through the Golgi to cell surface to present tumor-associated peptides to CD8+ T-cells.

The Role of MHC Antigens in T- and NK-Cell-Mediated Immunity

B lymphocytes are antibody producing cells capable of recognizing three-dimensional antigenic determinants on soluble native proteins, while T cells via T-cell receptor (TCR) recognize antigenic epitopes as linear peptide fragments bound to molecules of MHC complex on the surface of antigen-presenting cell (APC). Hence, antigen recognition by T lymphocytes is a tri-molecular interaction with APC that involves TCR expressed on the membrane of T cells and the anti-genic peptide bound to MHC molecule on the surface of APC (see Fig. 1.1). This interaction is influenced by MHC polymorphism within the residues located in the peptide-binding groove. The binding affinity between the peptide-binding site (TCR) and the pockets in the MHC binding groove is crucial for antigen recognition (Garbi et al. 2000). Therefore, the T-cell activation is restricted by specificity of the antigenic peptide and MHC allele. In addition, this process also requires co-stimulatory molecules without which this interaction will not lead to antigen-specific immune reaction.

Natural Killer (NK) cells belong to the lymphocyte lineage (Wang et al. 1998) and have important functions in both innate and acquired immune response. These cells display cytotoxic activity "in vitro" against a variety of tumor cells (Trinchieri 1989). Unlike B and T cells, NK cells do not have gene rearrangements of antigen-specific receptors (such as the TCR and BCR) (Long and Wagtmann 1997). An inverse correlation between tumor MHC class I expression and susceptibility to NK lysis has been established in a variety of cancers. Thus, loss of tumor MHC class I expression would render malignant cells susceptible NK-cell-mediated lysis ("missing self" hypothesis) (Ljunggren and Karre 1990). Furthermore, the ability of NK cells to acquire inhibitory receptors against self-HLA molecules has been described during NK cell maturation. Therefore, NK cells lyse target cells with total MHC loss or with very low level of expression of these molecules (Long 2002), a common event in transformed or virus-infected cells (Garrido et al. 1997; Ploegh 1998). NK cells are now recognized to express a repertoire of activating and inhibitory receptors, the physiological ratio of which is in equilibrium to ensure self-tolerance while allowing efficacy against assaults such as signs of infection, transformation, or stress (Lanier 2005; Orr and Lanier 2010; Vivier et al. 2011). NK cells recognize the density of different cell surface molecules that are expressed on the membrane of target cells. A combination of these different signals establishes the quality and the intensity of the NK-cell response. However, there are still many unanswered questions regarding NK-cell activation and function. The precise mechanisms of NK cell development and homeostasis are actively being investigated. Accumulating evidence in mice and humans suggests that, like the B and T cells of the adaptive immune system, NK cells are educated during development, possess antigen-specific receptors, undergo clonal expansion during infection and generate long-lived memory cells (Sun and Lanier 2011).

Mechanisms of Cancer Immune Escape

Currently there are many ongoing studies providing new experimental evidence that supports the cancer immunosurveillance concept first proposed by Burnet and Thomas (Burnet 1957). In the past two decades many studies have focused on trying to define the molecular basis of tumor escape mechanisms (Ahmad et al. 2004; Rivoltini et al. 2005; Vesely et al. 2011). Examples of different immune escape mechanisms are presented in Table 1.1.

It is also known that tumors may directly or indirectly inhibit the development of antitumor responses. Immunosurveillance is the protective function of the host performed by the immune system which preferably takes place at early stages of malignant transformation. However, the immune system through its continuous interaction with the tumor, can edit the immunogenicity of the tumor, resulting in the appearance of less immunogenic variants. Thus, the immune system has a dual nature; it helps to prevent tumor progression in early stages and promotes the selection of less immunogenic variants. This process is known as "cancer immunoediting"

Table 1.1 Various types of cancer immune escape mechanisms

Mechanisms	References
Loss of tumor antigen expression	Jager et al. (1996), Berset et al. (2001), Khong et al. (2004)
Defects in antigen-processing and presentation pathways: Loss of major histocompatibility complex (MHC) class I molecules and/or β2m. Loss of APM molecules: TAP1, LMP2, LMP7, and tapasin	Restifo et al. (1996), Marincola et al. (2000), Seliger et al. (2001), Meissner et al. (2005), Aptsiauri et al. (2007), Garrido et al. (2010)
Resistance of tumor cells to IFN-γ or IFN-α/β through either mutation or epigenetic silencing of genes encoding the IFN-γ receptor signaling components (IFNGR1, IFNGR2, JAK1, JAK2, and STAT1)	Kaplan et al. (1998), Dunn et al. (2005), Rodriguez et al. (2007), Respa et al. (2011)
Tumor-derived immunosuppressive factors that inhibit effector immune cell functions: Transforming growth factor-β (TGF-β); IL-10 Vascular endothelial growth factor (VEGF) that has an inhibitory effect on dendritic cells Metabolic enzymes such as indoleamine 2,3 dioxygenase (IDO) and arginase, that can locally inhibit immune responses by depleting amino acids essential for anabolic metabolism of T cells Gangliosides, soluble MICA Factors that recruit regulatory cells which generate an immunosuppressive microenvironment: IL-4, IL-13, GM-CSF, IL-1β, VEGF, or PGE2 Tumor-derived factors that inhibit DC function Colony-stimulating factors, IL-1β, VEGF, or PGE2 that increase an accumulation of MDSCs	Aruga et al. (1997), Gabrilovich et al. (1998), Khong and Restifo (2002), Uyttenhove et al. (2003), Terabe and Berzofsky (2004), Wrzesinski et al. (2007), Villablanca et al. (2010), Herber et al. (2010)
Mechanisms that provide tumors with the ability to escape immune destruction Upregulating inhibitors of apoptosis (Bcl-XL, FLIP) Expressing inhibitory cell surface molecules that directly kill cytotoxic T cells (PD-L1, FasL) Release of pro-apoptotic factors: TRAIL receptor, DR5, and Fas B7-H1 (PD-L1); that inhibit local antitumor T cell responses	Kataoka et al. (1998), Catlett-Falcone et al. (1999), Hinz et al. (2000), Shin et al. (2001), Dong et al. (2002), Takahashi et al. (2006), Zou et al. (2007)
Mechanisms that prevent tumor cell recognition by NK cells or CTLs: Loss of ligands for NK cell effector molecules (as NKG2D) Secretion by tumor of soluble ligands (as NKG2D) for effectors molecules that block T-cell and NK-cell function Inhibition of NK cells and CTLs through tumor cell expression of HLA-E or HLA-G Lack of expression of co-stimulatory molecules on malignant cells that can lead to failure of recognition of tumor antigens by T cells and suboptimal activation of NK cells Signaling defects through TCR: decreased expression of CD3ζ or tyrosine kinases	Aoe et al. (1995), Groh et al. (2002), Schultze and Nadler (2003), Carosella et al. (2003), Tripathi and Agrawal (2006), Derre et al. (2006), Stern-Ginossar et al. (2008)

(continued)

Table 1.1 (continued)

Mechanisms	References
The accumulation of regulatory cells decrease antitumor response through:	Sakaguchi et al. (2001), Terabe and Berzofsky (2004), Vesely et al. (2011)
Release of immunosuppressive cytokines, including IL-10 and TGF-β	
Altering the nutrient content of the microenvironment	
Inhibit effectors T cells through expression of CTLA-4 and PD-L1	
IL-2 consumption	
Recruitment and polarization of MDSCs from myeloid precursors that can block T cell function by expressing TGF- , ARG1, iNOS, and IDO	Vesely et al. (2011)

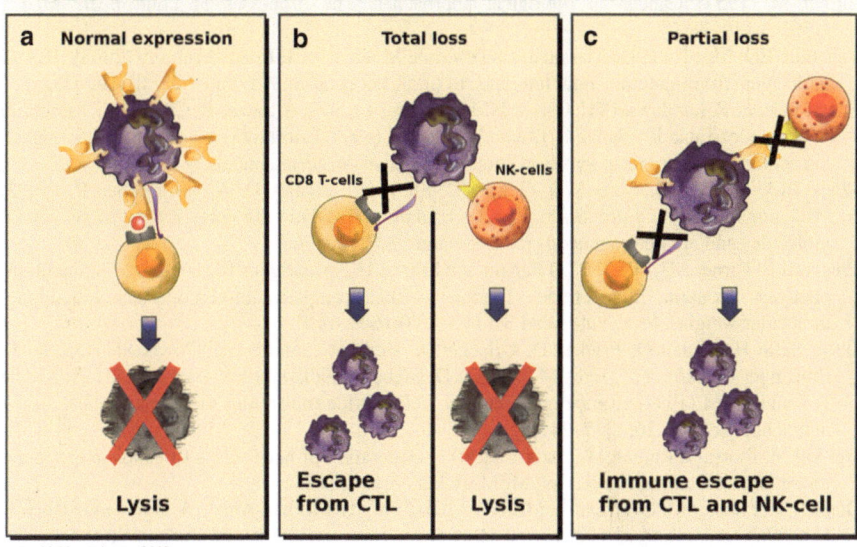

David Díez Cabrera. 2012

Fig. 1.2 Recognition of tumor cells by lymphocytes. (**a**) Cytotoxic T-cells (CTL) recognize tumor-associated antigenic peptide in complex with MHC class I complex leading to tumor cell lysis. (**b**) Total loss of MHC class I molecules on tumor cell provides a route of cancer immune escape from CTL, but renders tumor cells susceptible to NK-cell mediated lysis. (**c**) Immune escape from both CTL and NK cells associated with partial loss or low expression of MHC class I antigens

(Dunn et al. 2002; Schreiber et al. 2011). Later in this review we discuss data obtained by our group that support this hypothesis.

Altered HLA class I expression, as an important route of cancer immune escape, may have significant implications for the induction of antitumor cellular immunity. Figure 1.2 demonstrates possible scenarios of tumor cell recognition and elimination by T-cells or NK cells when HLA class I is either completely absent or shows abnormal level of expression.

References

Ahmad M, Rees RC, Ali SA (2004) Escape from immunotherapy: possible mechanisms that influence tumor regression/progression. Cancer Immunol Immunother 53:844–854

Amerik AY, Hochstrasser M (2004) Mechanism and function of deubiquitinating enzymes. Biochim Biophys Acta 1695(1–3):189–207

Aoe T, Okamoto Y, Saito T (1995) Activated macrophages induce structural abnormalities of the T-cell receptor-CD3 complex. J Exp Med 181(5):1881–1886

Aptsiauri N, Cabrera T, Garcia-Lora A, Lopez-Nevot MA, Ruiz-Cabello F, Garrido F (2007) MHC class I antigens and immune surveillance in transformed cells. Int Rev Cytol 256:139–189

Aruga A, Aruga E, Tanigawa K, Bishop DK, Sondak VK, Chang AE (1997) Type 1 versus type 2 cytokine release by V beta T cell subpopulations determines in vivo anti-tumor reactivity—IL-10 mediates a suppressive role. J Immunol 159(2):664–673

Berset M, Cerottini JP, Guggisberg D, Romero P, Burri F, Rimoldi D, Panizzon RG (2001) Expression of Melan-A/MART-1 antigen as a prognostic factor in primary cutaneous melanoma. Int J Cancer 95(1):73–77

Burnet M (1957) Cancer—a biological approach.1. The processes of control. Br Med J 1(5022):779–786

Carosella ED, Moreau P, Le Maoult J, Le Discorde M, Dausset J, Rouas-Freiss N (2003) HLA-G molecules: from maternal-fetal tolerance to tissue acceptance. Adv Immunol 81:199–252

Catlett-Falcone R, Landowski TH, Oshiro MM, Turkson J, Levitzki A, Savino R, Ciliberto G, Moscinski L, Fernández-Luna JL, Nuñez G, Dalton WS, Jove R (1999) Constitutive activation of Stat3 signaling confers resistance to apoptosis in human U266 myeloma cells. Immunity 10(1):105–115

Chicz RM, Urban RG, Lane WS, Gorga JC, Stern LJ, Vignali DAA, Strominger JL (1992) Predominant naturally processed peptides bound to HLA-DR1 are derived from MHC-related molecules and are heterogeneous in size. Nature 358:764–768

Cresswel P, Turner MJ, Jl S (1973) Papain-solubilized HL-A antigens from cultured human lymphocytes contain 2 peptide fragments—(histocompatibility-glycoproteins-membrane-molecular weight). Proc Natl Acad Sci U S A 70:1603–1607

De la Salle H, Hanau D, Fricker D, Urlacher A, Kelly A, Salamero J, Powis SH, Donato L, Bausinger H, Laforet M, Jeras M, Spehner D, Bieber T, Falkenrodt A, Cazenave JP, Trowsdale J, Tongio MM (1994) Homozygous human TAP peptide transporter mutation in HLA class-I deficiency. Science 265:237–241

Del Val M, Iborra S, Ramos M, Lazaro S (2011) Generation of MHC class I ligands in the secretory and vesicular pathways. Cell Mol Life Sci 68:1543–1552

Derre L, Corvaisier M, Charreau B, Moreau A, Godefroy E, Moreau-Aubry A, Jotereau F, Gervois N (2006) Expression and release of HLA-E by melanoma cells and melanocytes: Potential impact on the response of cytotoxic effector cells. J Immunol 177(5):3100–3107

Dong H, Strome SE, Salomao DR, Tamura H, Hirano F, Flies DB, Roche PC, Lu J, Zhu G, Tamada K, Lennon VA, Celis E, Chen L (2002) Tumor-associated B7-H1 promotes T-cell apoptosis: a potential mechanism of immune evasion. Nat Med 8(8):793–800

Dunn GP, Bruce AT, Ikeda H, Old LJ, Schreiber RD (2002) Cancer immunoediting: from immunosurveillance to tumor escape. Nat Immunol 3(11):991–998

Dunn GP, Sheehan KCF, Old LJ, Schreiber RD (2005) IFN unresponsiveness in LNCaP cells due to the lack of JAK1 gene expression. Cancer Res 65(8):3447–3453

Falk K, Rotzschke O, Stevanovic S, Jung G, Rammensee HG (1991) Allele-specific motifs revealed by sequencing of self-peptides eluted from MHC molecules. Nature 351:290–296

Gabrilovich D, Ishida T, Oyama T, Ran S, Kravtsov V, Nadaf S, Carbone DP (1998) Vascular endothelial growth factor inhibits the development of dendritic cells and dramatically affects the differentiation of multiple hematopoietic lineages in vivo. Blood 92(11):4150–4166

Garbi N, Tan P, Diehl AD, Chambers BJ, Ljunggren HG, Momburg F, Hammerling GJ (2000) Impaired immune responses and altered peptide repertoire in tapasin-deficient mice. Nat Immunol 1:234–238

Garrido F, Algarra I, García-Lora AM (2010) The escape of cancer from T lymphocytes: immunoselection of MHC class I loss variants harboring structural-irreversible "hard" lesions. Cancer Immunol Immunother 59(10):1601–1606

Garrido F, Ruiz-Cabello F, Cabrera T, Perez-Villar JJ, LopezBotet M, Duggan-Keen M, Stern PL (1997) Implications for immunosurveillance of altered HLA class I phenotypes in human tumours. Immunol Today 18:89–95

Geraghty DE (1993) Structure of the HLA class-I region and expression of its resident genes. Curr Opin Immunol 5:3–7

Goodfellow PN, Jones EA, Vanheyningen V, Solomon E, Bobrow M, Miggiano V, Bodmer WF (1975) Beta-2-microglobulin gene is on chromosome-15 and not in HL-A region. Nature 254:267–269

Grandea AG, Golovina TN, Hamilton SE, Sriram V, Spies T, Brutkiewicz RR, Harty JT, Eisenlohr LC, Van Kaer L (2000) Impaired assembly yet normal trafficking of MHC class I molecules in tapasin mutant mice. Immunity 13:213–222

Grandea AG, Van Kaer L (2001) Tapasin: an ER chaperone that controls MHC class I assembly with peptide. Trends Immunol 22:194–199

Groh V, WuJ YC, Spies T (2002) Tumour-derived soluble MIC ligands impair expression of NKG2D and T-cell activation. Nature 419:734–738

Herber DL, Cao W, Nefedova Y, Novitskiy SV, Nagaraj S, Tyurin VA, Corzo A, Cho HI, Celis E, Lennox B, Knight SC, Padhya T, McCaffrey TV, McCaffrey JC, Antonia S, Fishman M, Ferris RL, Kagan VE, Gabrilovich DI (2010) Lipid accumulation and dendritic cell dysfunction in cancer. Nat Med 16(8):880–886

Hinz S, Trauzold A, Boenicke L, Sandberg C, Beckmann S, Bayer E, Walczak H, Kalthoff H, Ungefroren H (2000) Bcl-X-L protects pancreatic adenocarcinoma cells against CD95-and TRAIL-receptor-mediated apoptosis. Oncogene 19(48):5477–5486

Jager E, Ringhoffer M, Karbach J, Arand M, Oesch F, Knuth A (1996) Inverse relation-ship of melanocyte differentiation antigen expression in melanoma tissues and CD8(+) cytotoxic-T-cell responses: evidence for immunoselection of antigen-loss variants in vivo. Int J Cancer 66(4):470–476

Kaplan DH, Shankaran V, Dighe AS, Stockert E, Aguet M, Old LJ, Schreiber RD (1998) Demonstration of an interferon gamma-dependent tumor surveillance system in immunocompetent mice. Proc Natl Acad Sci U S A 95(13):7556–7561

Kataoka T, Schroter M, Hahne M, Schneider P, Irmler M, Thome M, Froelich CJ, Tschopp J (1998) FLIP prevents apoptosis induced by death receptors but not by perforin/granzyme B, chemotherapeutic drugs, and gamma irradiation. J Immunol 161(8):3936–3942

Khong HT, Restifo NP (2002) Natural selection of tumor variants in the generation of "tumor escape" phenotypes. Nat Immunol 3(11):999–1005

Khong HT, Wang QJ, Rosenberg SA (2004) Identification of multiple antigens recognized by tumor-infiltrating lymphocytes from a single patient: tumor escape by antigen loss and loss of MHC expression. J Immunother 27(3):184–190

Lanier LL (2005) NK cell recognition. Annu Rev Immunol 23:225–274

Lehner PJ, Surman MJ, Cresswell P (1998) Soluble tapasin restores MHC class I expression and function in the tapasin-negative cell line.220. Immunity 8:221–231

Lehner PJ, Trowsdale J (1998) Antigen presentation: coming out gracefully. Curr Biol 8(17):R605–R608

Ljunggren HG, Karre K (1990) In search of the missing self—MHC molecules and NK cell recognition. Immunol Today 11(7):237–244

Long EO (2002) Tumor cell recognition by natural killer cells. Semin Cancer Biol 12(1):57–61

Long EO, Wagtmann N (1997) Natural killer cell receptors. Curr Opin Immunol 9(3):344–350

Lorente E, Garcia R, Lopez D (2011) Allele-dependent processing pathways generate the endogenous human leukocyte antigen (HLA) class I peptide repertoire in transporters associated with antigen processing (TAP)-deficient Cells. J Biol Chem 286:38054–38059

Marincola FM, Jaffee EM, Hicklin DJ, Ferrone S (2000) Escape of human solid tumors from T-cell recognition: molecular mechanisms and functional significance. Adv Immunol 74:181–273

Meissner M, Reichert TE, Kunkel M, Gooding W, Whiteside TL, Ferrone S, Seliger B (2005) Defects in the human leukocyte antigen class I antigen-processing machinery in head and neck squamous cell carcinoma: association with clinical outcome. Clin Cancer Res 11(7):2552–2560

Merzougui N, Kratzer R, Saveanu L, van Endert P (2011) A proteasome-dependent, TAP-independent pathway for cross-presentation of phagocytosed antigen. EMBO Rep 12:1257–1264

Monaco JJ (1992) A molecular-model of MHC class-I-restricted antigen processing. Immunol Today 13:173–178

Orr MT, Lanier LL (2010) Natural killer cell education and tolerance. Cell 142:847–856

Pickart CM, Cohen RE (2004) Proteasomes and their kin: proteases in the machine age. Nat Rev Mol Cell Biol 5:177–187

Ploegh HL (1998) Viral strategies of immune evasion. Science 280(5361):248–253

Respa A, Bukur J, Ferrone S, Pawelec G, Zhao Y, Wang E, Marincola FM, Seliger B (2011) Association of IFN-gamma signal transduction defects with impaired HLA class I antigen processing in melanoma cell lines. Clin Cancer Res 17(9):2668–2678

Restifo NP, Marincola FM, Kawakami Y, Taubenberger J, Yannelli JR, Rosenberg SA (1996) Loss of functional beta(2)-microglobulin in metastatic melanomas from five patients receiving immunotherapy. J Natl Cancer Inst 88(2):100–108

Rivoltini L, Canese P, Huber V, Iero M, Pilla L, Valenti R, Fais S, Lozupone F, Casati C, Castelli C, Parmiani G (2005) Escape strategies and reasons for failure in the interaction between tumour cells and the immune system: how can we tilt the balance towards immune-mediated cancer control? Expert Opin Biol Ther 5(4):463–476

Robinson J, Mistry K, McWilliam H, Lopez R, Parham P, Marsh SGE (2011) The IMGT/HLA database. Nucleic Acids Res 39(Database issue):D1171–D1176

Rodriguez T, Mendez R, Del Campo A, Jimenez P, Aptsiauri N, Garrido F, Ruiz-Cabello F (2007) Distinct mechanisms of loss of IFN-gamma mediated HLA class I inducibility in two melanoma cell lines. BMC Cancer 7:34

Rotzschke O, Falk K, Deres K, Schild H, Norda M, Metzger J, Jung G, Rammensee HG (1990) Isolation and analysis of naturally processed viral peptides as recognized by cytotoxic T-cells. Nature 348:252–254

Sakaguchi S, Sakaguchi N, Shimizu J, Yamazaki S, Sakihama T, Itoh M, Kuniyasu Y, Nomura T, Toda M, Takahashi T (2001) Immunologic tolerance maintained by CD25+ CD4+ regulatory T cells: their common role in controlling autoimmunity, tumor immunity, and transplantation tolerance. Immunol Rev 182:18–32

Seliger B, Ritz U, Abele R, Bock M, Tampe R, Sutter G, Drexler I, Huber C, Ferrone S (2001) Immune escape of melanoma: first evidence of structural alterations in two distinct components of the MHC class I antigen processing pathway. Cancer Res 61(24):8647–8650

Schreiber RD, Old LJ, Smyth MJ (2011) Cancer immunoediting: integrating immunity's roles in cancer suppression and promotion. Science 331(6024):1565–1570

Schultze JL, Nadler LM (2003) Lack of sufficient B7 expression as a tumor escape mechanism: implications for immunotherapy. In: Ochoa AC (ed) Mechanisms of tumor escape from the immune response. Taylor & Francis, London, pp 66–93

Shepherd JC, Schumacher TNM, Ashtonrickardt PG, Imaeda S, Ploegh HL, Janeway CA, Tonegawa S (1993) TAP1-dependent peptide translocation in-vitro is ATP-dependent and peptide selective. Cell 74(3):577–584

Shin EC, Ahn JM, Kim CH, Choi Y, Ahn YS, Kim H, Kim SJ, Park JH (2001) IFN-gamma induces cell death in human hepatoma cells through a trail/death receptor-mediated apoptotic pathway. Int J Cancer 93(2):262–268

Stern LJ, Wiley DC (1994) Antigenic peptide binding by class-I and class-II histocompatibility proteins. Structure 2:245–251

Stern-Ginossar N, Gur C, Biton M, Horwitz E, Elboim M, Stanietsky N, Mandelboim M, Mandelboim O (2008) Human microRNAs regulate stress-induced immune responses mediated by the receptor NKG2D. Nat Immunol 9:1065–1073

Sun JC, Lanier LL (2011) NK cell development, homeostasis and function: parallels with CD8(+) T cells. Nat Rev Immunol 11(10):645–657

Takahashi H, Feuerhake F, Kutok JL, Monti S, Dal Cin P, Neuberg D, Aster JC, Shipp MA (2006) FAS death domain deletions and cellular FADD-like interleukin 1 beta converting enzyme inhibitory protein (long) overexpression: alternative mechanisms for deregulating the extrinsic apoptotic pathway in diffuse large B-cell lymphoma subtypes. Clin Cancer Res 12(11 Pt 1):3265–3271

Terabe M, Berzofsky JA (2004) Immunoregulatory T cells in tumor immunity. Curr Opin Immunol 16(2):157–162

Townsend A, Bodmer H (1989) Antigen recognition by class-I restricted lymphocyte-T. Annu Rev Immunol 7:601–624

Townsend A, Elliott T, Cerundolo V, Foster L, Barber B, Tse A (1990) Assembly of MHC class-I molecules analyzed in vitro. Cell 62:285–295

Trinchieri G (1989) Biology of natural-killer cells. Adv Immunol 47:187–376

Tripathi P, Agrawal S (2006) Non-classical HLA-G antigen and its role in the cancer progression. Cancer Invest 24(2):178–186

Uyttenhove C, Pilotte L, Theate I, Stroobant V, Colau D, Parmentier N, Boon T, Van den Eynde BJ (2003) Evidence for a tumoral immune resistance mechanism based on tryptophan degradation by indoleamine 2,3-dioxygenase. Nat Med 9(10):1269–1274

Van Kaer L, Ashtonrickardt PG, Ploegh HL, Tonegawa S (1992) TAP1 mutant mice are deficient in antigen presentation, surface class-I molecules, and CD4-8+ T-cells. Cell 71:1205–1214

Vesely MD, Kershaw MH, Schreiber RD, Smyth MJ (2011) Natural innate and adaptive immunity to cancer. Annu Rev Immunol 29:235–271

Villablanca EJ, Raccosta L, Zhou D, Fontana R, Maggioni D, Negro A, Sanvito F, Ponzoni M, Valentinis B, Bregni M, Prinetti A, Steffensen KR, Sonnino S, Gustafsson JA, Doglioni C, Bordignon C, Traversari C, Russo V (2010) Tumor-mediated liver X receptor-alpha activation inhibits CC chemokine receptor-7 expression on dendritic cells and dampens antitumor responses. Nat Med 16(1):98–105

Vivier E, Raulet DH, Moretta A, Caligiuri MA, Zitvogel L, Lanier LL, Yokoyama WM, Ugolini S (2011) Innate or adaptive immunity? The example of natural killer cells. Science 331(6013):44–49

Wang M, Ellison CA, Gartner JG, HayGlass KT (1998) Natural killer cell depletion fails to influence initial CD4 T cell commitment in vivo in exogenous antigen-stimulated cytokine and antibody responses. J Immunol 160(3):1098–1105

Wrzesinski SH, Wan YY, Flavell RA (2007) Transforming growth factor-beta and the immune response: implications for anticancer therapy. Clin Cancer Res 13(18 Pt 1):5262–5270

Zou W, Chen S, Liu X, Yue P, Sporn MB, Khuri FR, Sun SY (2007) c-FLIP downregulation contributes to apoptosis induction by the novel synthetic triterpenoid methyl-2-cyano-3,12-dioxooleana-1,9-dien-28-oate (CDDO-Me) in human lung cancer cells. Cancer Biol Ther 6(10):1614–1620

Chapter 2
HLA Class I Expression in Human Cancer

Altered HLA Class I Expression in Malignant Cells

Loss or down-regulation of HLA class I antigens in tumor cells has been frequently observed in a variety of human malignancies and it represents an important cancer immune escape mechanism (Garrido et al. 1997a; Marincola et al. 2000; Campoli et al. 2002; Chang et al. 2005; Aptsiauri et al. 2007). Viruses use similar mechanism to avoid recognition and elimination by the immune system (Ploegh 1998). The first description of MHC class I loss was done in a mouse model (Gardener lymphoma) in Dr. Festenstein laboratory in 1976 (Garrido et al. 1976a, b). The production and characterization of monoclonal antibodies against HLA molecules (Barnstable et al. 1978) made possible to analyze HLA expression in human cell lines and solid tumors. At first, the reported percentage of HLA class I loss was low (10–30 %) (Garrido et al. 1993), since only monomorphic monoclonal antibodies (recognizing an epitope common to all HLA class I molecules) were available at that time. These studies were able to detect only total loss of tumor HLA class I expression and due to low incidence these findings did not attract much attention and were not considered to be significant. Later on, with the appearance of more specific monoclonal antibodies (anti-locus-A, -B and anti-allele-specific antibodies), which recognize polymorphic portions of these molecules, the incidence of HLA altered expression in cancer has been found to be much higher, increasing the relevance of these defects in the immune response against tumor. Using a broad panel of monoclonal antibodies on cryostat tumor tissue sections these alterations have been found in 60–90 % of tumors depending on the histological type of cancer (Blades et al. 1995; Cabrera et al. 1996, 1998, 2000; Koopman et al. 2000; Kageshita et al. 2005). Unfortunately, the number of available allele-specific monoclonal antibodies is still limited. Therefore, the true percentage of HLA class I defects, especially allelic losses, may perhaps be much higher in different types of malignancy.

Thus, early studies using immunohistological analysis of different tumors showed a very low frequency of allelic loss. However, with the arrival of other techniques, such as the study of microsatellites to detect loss of heterozygosity

N. Aptsiauri et al., *MHC Class I Antigens In Malignant Cells: Immune Escape and Response to Immunotherapy*, SpringerBriefs in Cancer Research 6, DOI 10.1007/978-1-4614-6543-0_2, © Teresa Cabrera 2013

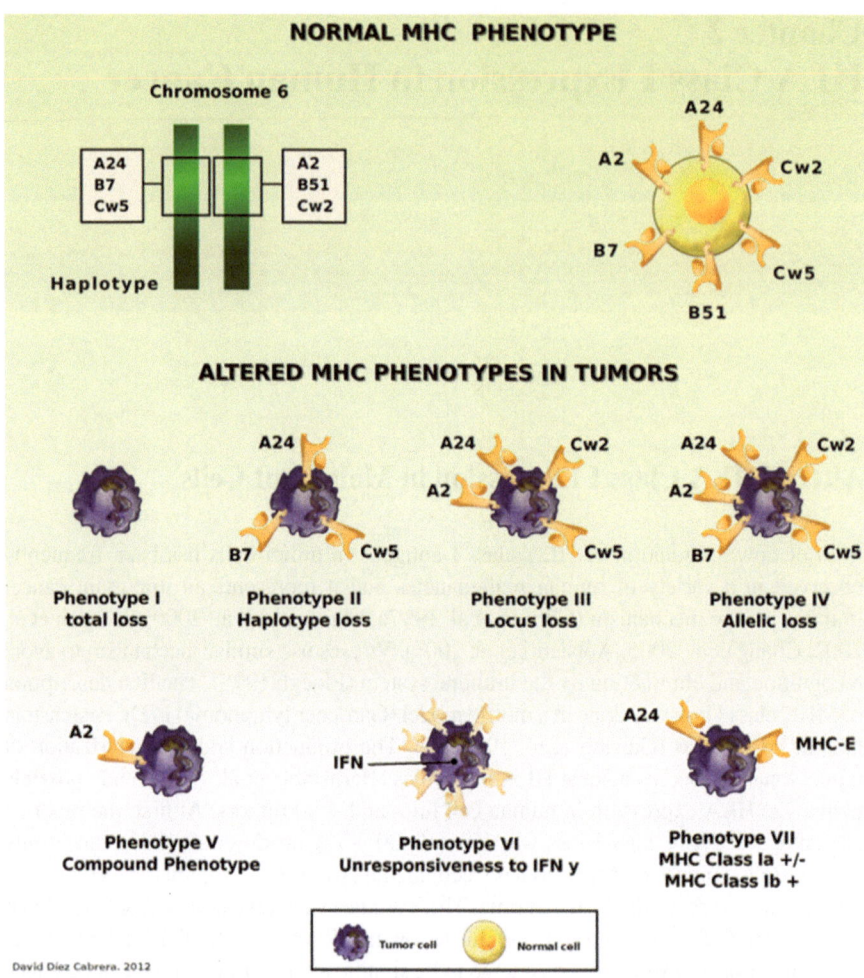

Fig. 2.1 Altered MHC class I phenotypes found in human tumors. Two copies of the genes coding for HLA class I heavy chain are located in chromosome 6. Each cell normally expresses six HLA class I alleles (two HLA-A, two HLA-B, and two HLA-C). HLA class I molecules can be totally or partially absent from tumor cells (Phenotype I to Phenotype V). In some cases tumor cells do not change class I expression after treatment with IFN-γ (Phenotype VI). Some tumor cells express aberrant HLA-E molecules together with low expression of HLA-A, -B, or -C classical class I antigens (Phenotype VII)

(LOH) on chromosome 6, it has been shown that LOH (haplotype loss) is the most frequent alteration of class I expression (Feenstra et al. 2000; Koopman et al. 2000; Maleno et al. 2002, 2004a, 2006). This alteration is caused by various defects in the HLA genomic region (short arm of chromosome 6, 6p21), including chromosomal dysfunction, mitotic recombination, and genetic conversion.

Many years of analysis of HLA expression in human tumors and tumor cell lines permitted us to classify HLA class I alterations in seven phenotypes according to the cell surface expression pattern (Garcia-Lora et al. 2003) (see Fig. 2.1):

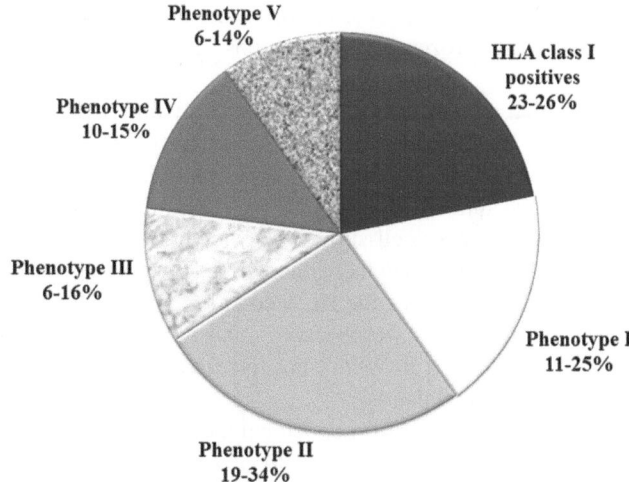

Fig. 2.2 Distribution of HLA class I phenotypes among different types of cancer

Phenotype I: Total loss of HLA class I molecules
Phenotype II: Loss of an HLA class I haplotype
Phenotype III: Loss of an HLA class I locus
Phenotype IV: HLA class I allelic loss
Phenotype V: Compound phenotype
Phenotype VI: Failure to respond to interferon (IFN)
Phenotype VII: Low expression (down-regulation) of classical HLA molecules (Ia)
    with aberrant expression of non-classical HLA molecules (Ib)

Based on the results of tumor immunohistochemistry and molecular analysis many groups have investigated the frequency of various HLA class I altered phenotypes in different types of cancer. This information is important for better understanding of tissue-specific factors that influence HLA alterations during malignant transformation (Fig. 2.2).

Difficulties to Define HLA Class I Altered Phenotypes in Tumor Tissue

Immunohistochemistry remains to be the key method to analyze the expression of HLA molecules on tumor cells. We believe that accurate detection of HLA complex on tumor cell surface is fundamental, since it predetermines tumor cell recognition by both CTL and NK cells. However, in solid tumors this process has both technical difficulties and problems with the result interpretation, such as the following:

• Pathology laboratories routinely work with formalin-fixed paraffin-embedded tissues. However, the structure of HLA complex is very sensitive to this type of tissue processing and loses specific epitopes that are recognized by anti-HLA antibodies. Therefore, frozen tissues sections are the best choice for HLA analysis.

- Most antibodies that work in paraffin recognize only intra-cytoplasmic epitopes but not cell surface HLA complex, like HC-10 antibody which is directed against free intracellular heavy chain molecule. It is not unusual to see a positive immunolabeling of frozen tumor sections with HC-10 antibody and negative when W6/32 antibody (recognizes cell-surface HLA complex) is applied. This result usually indicates that there is a defect either in the assembly of HLA heavy chain with β2m or in the transport of the HLA complex to the cell surface (Cabrera et al. 2003b). In some cases we observed controversial results when we find HC-10-negative tumor nests in W6/32-positive tissue samples indicating tumor heterogeneity (unpublished data).

- Currently only limited number of monoclonal antibodies against HLA alleles is available (Garrido et al. 1997b). Monoclonal antibodies that recognize HLA alleles must be screened on frozen tissue sections, because some antibodies that are highly specific in cytotoxic assays do not react or display abnormal reactions in immunohistological techniques. To determine whether these antibodies are suitable, HLA typing of autologous patient PBMC should be done.

- Difficulties in the defining HLA class I expression phenotypes and in the interpretation of the intensity of immunohistochemical reactions analysis of HLA class I expression in tumor samples was discussed at the HLA expression & Cancer exercise of the 15th International Histocompatibility and Immunogenetics Workshop. Several participating laboratories were provided with the same tumor tissue material and antibodies. Bases on their final reports it was established that the intensity of immunohistochemical reactions was difficult to define since it varied significantly between the laboratories. Examples of immunohistological techniques with differences in the intensity of tumor cell staining are shown in Fig. 2.3.

- At the Workshop it was also discussed that partial HLA class I losses (haplotype loss, allelic loss, etc.) do not always correlate with the expected intensity of the immunolabeling. For instance, one might expect that tumors with LOH should show weaker staining due to the loss of the half of HLA genetic material. However, most of the workshop participants reported strongly positive W6/32 and β2m labeling of frozen section of tumor samples known to have LOH (unpublished data).

New techniques are currently used to study HLA class I alterations in tumor samples, including RT-PCR, microsatellite analysis for detection of LOH, DNA sequencing, and others. But none of them alone can give us a complete picture of HLA class I alterations in a tumor. For example, LOH tells us about a haplotype loss, but this tumor may also have other alterations, like a total loss of expression. Furthermore, in several tumors using tissue microdissection and real-time PCR we observed high levels of HLA-B locus-specific transcription, however, on the protein level we did not see cell surface expression of locus B (Fig. 2.4) (Carretero et al.

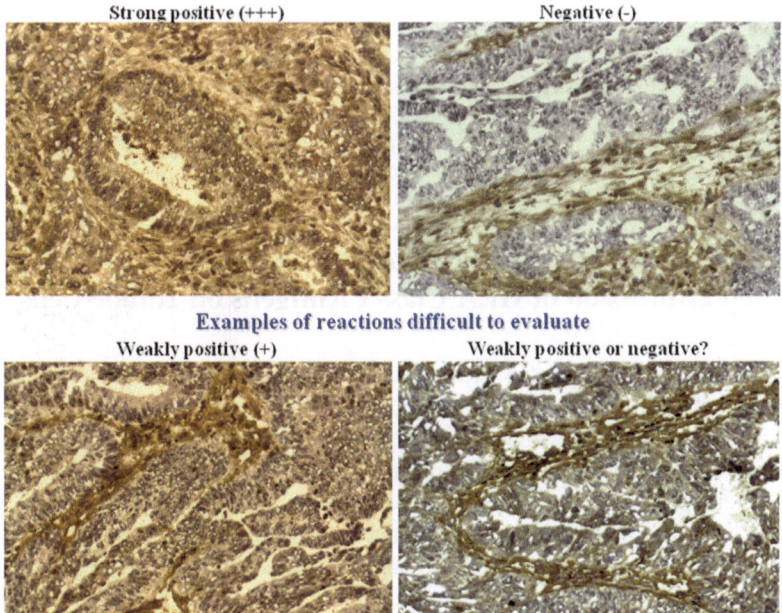

Fig. 2.3 Difficulties in the interpretation of the variations in the intensity of tumor HLA class I immunolabeling

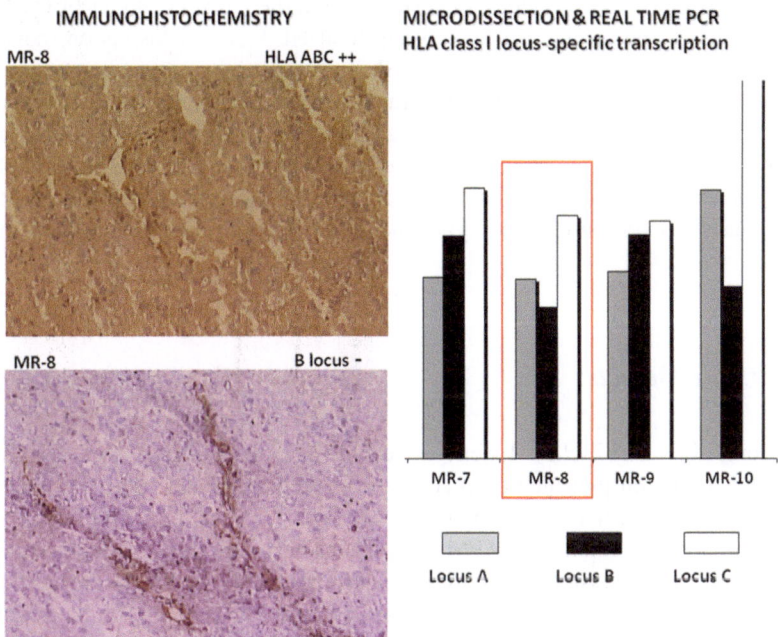

Fig. 2.4 High levels of HLA-B locus-specific transcription (*right panel*) and absence of tumor cell surface expression of locus B as shown by immunohistochemistry (*left panel*)

2008). In our experience, this is a good example demonstrating the frequent discrepancy between gene expression and cell surface protein expression of HLA class I molecules in tumor cells. We believe that in order to define HLA altered phenotypes it is essential to use a combination of all the existing techniques.

Reversible and Irreversible Molecular Defects Underlying Altered Expression of HLA Class I Antigens on Tumor Cells

From experimental work it is clear that the malignant behavior of a cancer cell depends not only on the level of tumor MHC class I expression, but also on the molecular mechanisms which cause alterations in the MHC class I expression. Generation of various tumor MHC phenotypes can occur at any step required for the protein synthesis, assembly, transport or expression on cell surface. These defects can occur at the genetic, epigenetic, transcriptional, and posttranscriptional levels and represent either regulatory abnormalities that can be recovered with cytokine treatment or more severe structural defects. Thus, MHC alterations can be classified into two main groups: reversible regulatory defects, and irreversible structural defects (Garrido et al. 2010). Although regulatory defects on transcriptional level are more common among various types of malignancy, the structural MHC defects may have profound implications in the T-cell mediated rejection of tumor cells in primary or metastatic lesions and in the outcome of cancer immunotherapy. When the mechanism underlying total HLA class I loss is on transcriptional level, the expression of surface HLA class I antigens can be reversed by cytokine treatment and T-cell based therapy can be successfully applied. However, peptide-based immunotherapy aimed at augmenting T-cell-specific tumor recognition may not be effective in case of irreversible damage of HLA genes. Therefore, development of an adequate diagnostic approach for precise identification of the HLA class I expression phenotype and underlying molecular mechanisms is central.

Reversible Defects

The reversible MHC class I deficiencies involve all levels of the MHC class I-restricted antigen presentation machinery on transcriptional level. They can be repaired, at least partially and in vitro, by cytokines (IFN-gamma, TNF-alpha). The IFN-mediated upregulation of APM components normally leads to enhanced MHC class I surface expression and improves antitumor CTL responses (Seliger et al. 2000; Martini et al. 2010). Thus, it represents a valuable strategy for the treatment of patients with APM deficiencies. However, in some cases, tumors remain insensitive to IFN treatment despite the lack of structural alterations in APM components, suggesting an impaired IFN signal transduction (Rodriguez et al. 2007).

Down-regulation of TAP1/2 and LMP2/7 gene has been demonstrated in different cell lines and tumor lesions (Cabrera et al. 2003a, c; Meissner et al. 2005). LMP7 down-regulation was found in correlation with the level of MHC class I expression in various human cancer cell lines (Yoon et al. 2000). A high frequency of LMP2, LMP7, and TAP1 down-regulation or loss was observed in tumor lesions and cell lines obtained from head and neck cancer patients, which could be reversed by IFN-gamma treatment (Meissner et al. 2005). Impaired expression of immunoproteasome subunits (Cabrera et al. 2003a, c; Miyagi et al. 2003) and tapasin (Cabrera et al. 2005) is involved in different types of HLA class I molecule loss in human colon cancer.

Epigenetic events associated with tumor development and cancer progression have been found to underlie changes in HLA and APM expression and activity. HLA class I gene hypermethylation leading to HLA loss has been demonstrated in various types of cancer. These alterations can be reversed in vitro with pharmacologic agents that induce DNA hypomethylation or inhibit histone deacetylation (Serrano et al. 2001).

Irreversible Alterations

Total loss of HLA class I expression is caused by various mutations and chromosomal defects involving genes encoding heavy chain or β2-microglobulin. HLA haplotype loss is one of the most frequent described phenotypes. This alteration is caused by the hemizygous loss of HLA-A, -B and -C alleles or by loss of one copy of chromosome 6 (Torres et al. 1996). This type of HLA class I alteration mechanism has been described in different types of malignancy, e.g., laryngeal tumor (Maleno et al. 2002), melanoma (Rodriguez et al. 2005), colorectal tumor (Maleno et al. 2004a), non-Hodgkin's lymphoma (Drénou et al. 2004), and pancreatic cancer (Ryschich et al. 2004). Allelic loss of single HLA alleles defines another HLA phenotype that is caused by a wide array of genetic defects including point mutations, frameshifts, or deletions (Jiménez et al. 2001).

LOH in chromosome 15 (β2m gene region) can be frequently detected in tumors (in 40 % of colon melanomas and laryngeal carcinomas and in 50 % of bladder carcinomas) (Maleno et al. 2011). This lesion in chromosome 15 may be unnoticed since tumor cells might have "normal" HLA class I pattern and it could represent one of the early events in malignant cells leading to generation of precommitted tumors to become HLA escape variants. LOH in chromosome 15 in tumors can be found more frequently than mutations in β2m gene.

HLA class I gene mutations include somatic recombination within class I genes (Browning et al. 1996), nonsense mutations (Koopman et al. 2000), missense mutations, deletions, and insertions (Lehmann et al. 1995; Serrano et al. 2000; Jiménez et al. 2001).

Mutations in β2m genes range from large deletions to single nucleotide deletions and mutations are distributed randomly among the genes (Restifo et al. 1996; Benitez et al. 1998; Feenstra et al. 1999; Paschen et al. 2003). A mutation hotspot located in the CT repeat region of exon 1 of the β2m gene has been proposed (Pérez et al. 1999) reflecting an increased genetic instability in this region in malignant cells. A summary of β2m mutations discovered in tumor cell lines and tumor specimens has been recently reviewed (Bernal et al. 2012). In most of the cases, two structural defects are necessary to produce the total loss of HLA class I on malignant cells: β2m mutation in one copy of the β2m gene and loss of the other copy associated with loss of heterozygosity (LOH) in chromosome 15 (Paschen et al. 2006).

Mutations in various APM components appear to be a rare event postulating that dysregulation rather than structural alterations is the major cause for aberrant APM component expression. TAP mutation associated with HLA class I loss was described in lung cancer (Chen et al. 1996) and in melanoma (Seliger et al. 2001).

Resistance to IFN-γ-mediated upregulation of HLA class I expression can be also a mechanism producing tumor escape variants. It is caused by defects in the Jak-STAT components of interferon (IFN)-mediated signaling pathway (Rodriguez et al. 2005; Seliger et al. 2008).

Correlation Between HLA Class I Defects and Cancer Progression in Humans

Despite the recent advances in the understanding of the role of HLA class I antigen expression in tumors, information regarding its prognostic value or its association with patient outcome remains controversial. There are a large number of publications describing a relationship between traditional pathologic criteria and/or patient survival and HLA class I expression, but the results are inconsistent. Down-regulation or low expression of MHC class I antigens has been demonstrated to have an important cancer prognostic value in various studies (Marincola et al. 2000; Chang et al. 2003; Powell et al. 2012). Morabito and coworkers (2009) observed that down-regulation of HLA class I expression in breast cancer has a significant association with adverse prognostic factors. Kaneko et al. (2011) reported that patients with preserved HLA class I expression have significantly better disease-free interval than those with loss of HLA class I. Down-regulation of HLA class I in rectal cancer has been associated with poor prognosis (Speetjens et al. 2008). On the other hand, loss of class I expression has been associated with good prognosis in breast carcinoma and non-small-cell lung cancer (Madjd et al. 2005; Ramnath et al. 2006).

At the same time, several studies have failed to show a correlation between HLA-expression and patient prognosis (Marincola et al. 2000; Chang et al. 2003; Powell et al. 2012). Normal expression of HLA class I in a non-small-cell lung cancer was associated with a favorable prognosis compared with the heterogeneous expression group, but no significant difference was observed between the normal expression and decreased expression groups (Hanagiri et al. 2012). Kikuchi et al. (2007) revealed down-regulation of HLA class I as an independent factor of poor prognosis in stage I patients, but not in late-stage patient. Two studies have found that total absence of HLA class I resulted in a favourable prognosis as compared to patients with low tumor HLA expression. One study describes that high expression of HLA class I in tumor cells associated with better prognosis as compared to the partial down-regulation of HLA class I (Watson et al. 2006), while another report proved totally opposite findings (Menon et al. 2002). Partial HLA class I loss has also been significantly associated with decreased 5-years overall survival in breast cancer (Kaneko et al. 2011).

We believe that the inconsistencies among these studies may be explained by various reasons:

- Most of the studies are done on paraffin-embedded tissue using monoclonal antibodies able to detect only total loss of expression. In addition, as we have explained above, these antibodies react with intracytoplasmic HLA molecules and do not interact with cell surface epitopes.
- In other studies, even though they analyze cryopreserved tissue, the use of monomorphic antibodies limits the detection only to a total loss of HLA class I; and it is currently recognized other types of HLA loss are also important.
- Differences in the techniques with different degree of sensitivity; as we discussed earlier in this review, the intensity of the immunolabeling is often difficult to evaluate.
- Some studies report poor prognosis to be associated with an "intermediate" HLA class I expression. In other publications "partial HLA class I loss" is named as a bad prognosis factor. The difference in terminology used to describe abnormal HLA expression creates certain confusion. It is not clear whether "intermediate" and "partial loss" refer to the intensity of the immunolabeling or they describe the loss of a particular locus or allele.
- Expression of non-classical molecules should be analysed and taken into account because of their importance for NK cell inhibition (Carosella et al. 2003).

We believe that the correlation between HLA expression and clinical outcome cannot be clearly defined without identification of the exact type of tumor HLA defects (which alleles are missing) in each patient, which would predict the ability of CTLs to recognize tumor-associated peptides. Tumor cells with total HLA loss are not recognized by CTL, but NK cells should be able to target them for elimination. Tumors with partial loss may evade both NK- and T-cell-mediated immune surveillance; if the allele responsible for peptide presentation is missing, the remaining allele can inhibit NK cells (see Fig. 1.2).

Role of HLA Class I Altered Expression in Resistance to Immunotherapy

Malignant transformation is characterized by accumulation of genetic alterations and by epigenetic aberrations in tumor cells leading to expression of atypical proteins called tumor-associated antigens (TAA). Recognition of TAA by HLA class I-restricted CD8+ T cells is fundamental for the detection and destruction of malignant cells (van der Bruggen et al. 1991). The discovery of TAA has changed the field of cancer treatment and introduced a new era of cancer immunotherapy aimed at increasing tumor immunogenicity and T-cell-mediated antitumor immunity. Unfortunately, while the new protocols of cancer immunotherapy increase the presence of tumor-specific T lymphocytes and/or demonstrated partial responses in patients with certain malignancies, they have not yet delivered significant clinical benefits, such as induction of tumor regression or increased disease-free survival (Rosenberg et al. 2004). The results of early clinical trials were not very promising, but with the introduction of adjuvants and implementation of more innovative monitoring and evaluation criteria (Response Evaluation Criteria in Solid Tumors, RECIST), the outcome of cancer immunotherapy protocols has improved (Klebanoff et al. 2011). In addition, our understanding of the molecular mechanisms of cancer immune escape and the role of complex interaction between tumor and the host has expanded leading to improved novel treatment approaches. In order to counteract immunosuppressive factors of tumor microenvironment novel strategies are being evaluated in both clinical and preclinical settings, including combination of immuno and chemotherapy, small-molecule targeted therapies, monoclonal antibodies used to block important immune checkpoint molecules, inhibitors of immune-suppression, etc. (Schlom 2012; Walter et al. 2012). Furthermore, initially, many vaccines were tested in patients with advanced metastatic disease treated with other types of cancer therapy. Clinical studies have shown that patients respond better to vaccines when they are treated at early disease stages with only limited previous clinical intervention (Schlom 2012).

Concurrent with US Food and Drug Administration (FDA) approval of the Sipuleucel-T vaccine (Kantoff et al. 2010), the first therapeutic cancer vaccine for the therapy of asymptomatic metastatic castrate-resistant prostate cancer, a broad spectrum of other cancer vaccines is at present being evaluated. Despite the obvious progress in cancer immunotherapy and vaccination, it is clear that, although it leads to a certain clinical improvement in some patients, no significant increase in cancer patient survival has been achieved yet.

Understanding of the possible causes of such poor clinical outcome has become very important for improvement of the existing cancer treatment modalities. In particular, the critical role of HLA class I antigens in the success of T cell based immunotherapy has led to a growing interest in investigating the expression and function of these molecules in metastatic cancer progression and, especially in response to immunotherapy.

As we discussed earlier in the review, the lack of tumor rejection is associated with multiple cancer immune escape mechanisms, including the loss or low expression of tumor HLA class I molecules. Absence of normal expression of HLA class I molecules

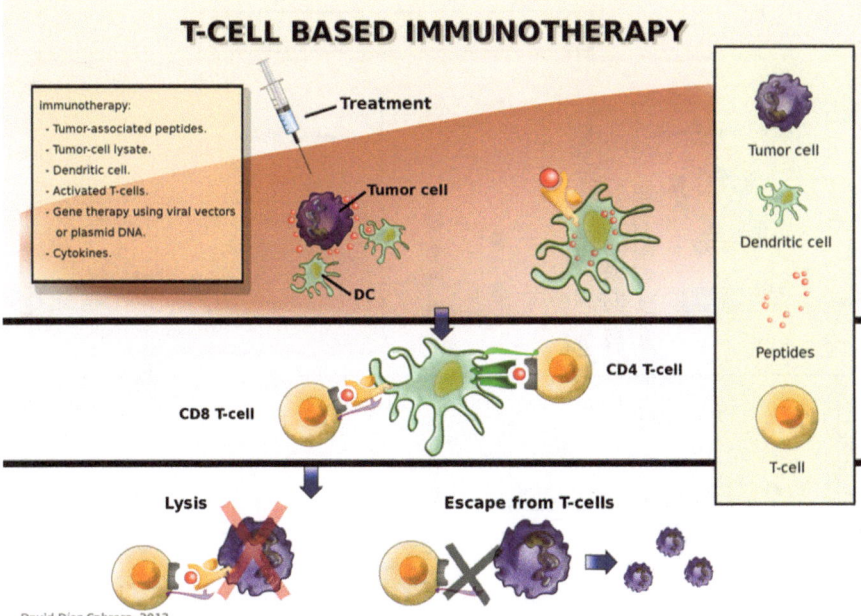

Fig. 2.5 Possible outcomes of cancer immunotherapy. The existing protocols of cancer immunotherapy are aimed at increasing the recognition of tumor cells by CD4 and CD8 T lymphocytes leading to tumor cell elimination by cytotoxic CD8 T cells. This recognition requires presentation of a tumor-associated peptide in a complex with HLA class I molecule to T cells. Therefore, absence or low expression of HLA molecules may diminish T-cell based antitumor immunity. T-cell based cancer immunotherapy induces upregulation of HLA class I in tumor cells with normal expression or with reversible HLA alterations leading to better recognition and elimination of cancer cells by CD8+ T-cell. Tumor cells escape from the immune system when HLA class I loss is caused by structural irreversible defects in HLA genes

on tumor cell surface expression obliterates TAA-peptide presentation to CTLs and leads to tumor progression. Therefore, immunotherapy aimed at increasing antitumor immune response may fail and not yield clinical benefit. Figure 2.5 shows that various types of T-cell-based cancer immunotherapy aimed are currently used in clinical setting. Each of them lead to activation of antitumor immune recognition mechanisms, starting with changes in tumor microenvironment, an increase in cytokine production, and induction of DC-mediated tumor-peptide presentation to both CD8 and CD4 T-cells. All this leads to HLA-restricted tumor cell recognition by CTLs and consequent elimination. However, if tumor cells lose normal HLA class I expression, they may escape T-cell recognition and proliferate. Therefore, the commonly observed MHC-I defects in tumors constitute a potential problem for T cell-based immunotherapy. In addition, the impact of MHC-I defects on the non-responding tumors is largely unknown and corrections of antigen presentation in these tumor types might result in much higher success rates (Lampen and van Hall 2011). Unfortunately, the majority of ongoing cancer immunotherapy clinical trials do not include tumor MHC class I expression analysis before or during the treatment, reducing the number of patient with potentially positive clinical response.

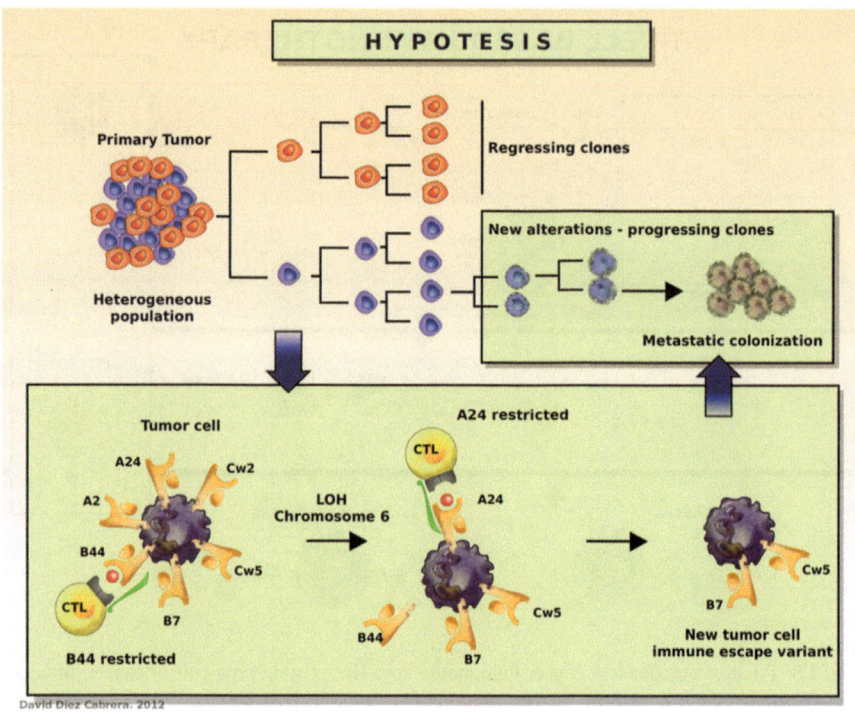

Fig. 2.6 HLA class I mediated immunoselection of tumor escape variants during cancer progression. Primary tumors consist of heterogeneous populations of cells that give rise to different cell clones undergoing immune selection. The combination of somatic evolution of genetically unstable tumor cells and immune selection during cancer development leads to the generation of tumor variants that have better survival properties. This selective pressure will lead to the expansion of new populations of cells with multiple defects capable of evading different immune responses. In this way, tumor cell with normal HLA class I expression are subjected to T-cell cytotoxic response restricted to an HLA class I allele (e.g., B44 restricted CTL reactivity). These cells are destroyed, but new HLA-negative clones appear due to additional alterations. LOH in chromosome 6 causes HLA haplotype loss and generation of B44-negative cell clones. These newly emerged clones are positive for HLA-A24 and CTL response is now A24-restricted leading to elimination of HLA-A24 positive malignant cells, but new tumor escape variants appear

The importance of monitoring tumor HLA class I expression is well illustrated by the report in which a longer overall survival in renal cell cancer was associated with immune responses to multiple tumor-associated peptides (TUMAPs) used for vaccination (Walter et al. 2012). They treated 96 HLA-A*02 RCC patients with peptides presented by HLA-A2 without previously analyzing tumor for HLA-A2 expression. We beleive, that pre-selection of patients with tumors expressing HLA-A2 for this clinicla trial would have improve the outcome of the therapy.

Moreover, accumulating evidence suggests that tumor cells that escape immune response during immunomodulating treatment have more dangerous metastatic phenotype due to accumulation of more profound genetic alterations (see Fig. 2.6). In this regard, the results that we have obtained recently in our laboratory support this theory.

HLA and Resistance to Immunotherapy in Melanoma and Bladder Cancer

We have studied different melanoma metastases from patients with mixed response to immunotherapy and several bladder tumors from patients treated with Bacillus Calmette-Guerin (BCG). We observed a strong correlation between tumor progression/recurrence and response to therapy with defects in tumor HLA class I expression and the nature of underlying mechanisms of these alterations (reversible or irreversible).

One melanoma patient developed several metastases after therapy with autologous tumor cell vaccine together and BCG (M-VAX), including three progressing and three regressing lesions. Another melanoma patient was treated first with interferon $\alpha 2b$ and later with M-VAX. We studied several progressing and regressing metastases obtained after each of the therapy modalities. All metastases showed HLA class I alterations. However, the progressing metastases developed additional and more profound defects in HLA class I expression.

All metastases from the first melanoma patient presented loss of heterozygosity (LOH) in chromosome 6. In addition, progressing metastases showed a weaker expression of HLA class I, loss of HLA-B locus, and LOH in chromosome 15 (Cabrera et al. 2007). None of the metastatic samples from the second melanoma patients showed LOH in chromosomes 6 or 15, although loss of HLA-B we detected in all the samples. Progressing metastases developed new defects in the HLA system after the therapy (Carretero et al. 2008). Quantitative expression analysis of HLA-A, B, and C genes on microdissected tumor areas demonstrated higher HLA expression in regressing than in progressing metastases (Carretero et al. 2012).

A comparative gene expression analysis of these 15 metastases (10 regressing and 5 progressing) obtained from mixed melanoma responders to different types of therapy allowed us to isolate genes differentially expressed in regressing and progressing lesions, with the majority of them being implicated in regulation of the immune response. Upregulation of antigen presentation and immune rejection pathways, including HLA-A, B, and C, antigen processing machinery (APM), interferon regulatory factor 1 (IRF-I), signal transducers and activators of transcription 1 (STAT-1), allograft inflammatory factor (AIF-l), granzymes, etc., were found in regressing metastases. In contrast, progressing metastases showed low transcription levels of genes involved in these pathways (Carretero et al. 2012). These data suggest that regressing tumors are under an acute immune rejection response. The molecular signature of tumor rejection in our case appeared to be similar to those described during allograft rejection, autoimmune disease, graft-versus-host disease and pathogen clearance.

We have also showed that BCG immunotherapy of bladder cancer induces selection of HLA class I-deficient tumor cells (Carretero et al. 2011). We performed a comparative analysis of HLA class I expression in recurrent bladder tumors in patients treated with mitomycin or BCG. HLA class I expression was studied in 18 bladder cancer patients in total. Among 13 patient treated with BCG, eight were relapse-free, while five patients developed recurrent tumors after the therapy. Five mitomycin-treated patients were used as controls. Both primary and recurrent tumors were studied. More profound alterations in HLA class I expression were found in post-BCG recurrent tumors than in pre-BCG lesions, whereas mitomycin treatment did not change the HLA class I expression pattern. Post-BCG recurrent tumors also showed a higher incidence of structural defects underlying altered HLA class I expression: 80 and 60 % of tumors showed (LOH) in chromosomes 6 and 15, whereas only 25 % of relapse-free patients had LOH in either chromosome.

A whole genome transcriptional analysis is also being carried in 13 primary bladder tumors obtained from six relapse-free patients and seven patients with relapse after several years of follow-up. Preliminary results showed that antigen presentation and interferon pathway genes are highly expressed in tumors from relapse-free patients versus patients with recurrence, which showed higher expression level of molecules associated with Th17 lymphocytes as compared to relapse-free patients. Patients without recurrence also showed higher expression of Th1-related molecules (unpublished data).

Our results show that tumors with irreversible alterations in HLA class I can escape the immune system despite immunotherapy. We suggest that tumors with reversible alterations will better response to immunotherapy by upregulation the antigen presentation machinery, leading to tumor cell recognition and elimination by T cells. In contrast, transformed cells bearing irreversible structural defects have low probability to have a positive response to immunomodulating treatment and will continue to grow. Therefore, expression of HLA class I alterations in tumor cells is a key factor to be considered during selection of immunotherapy strategy and is a biomarker to be monitored during treatment.

References

Aptsiauri N, Cabrera T, Mendez R, Garcia-Lora A, Ruiz-Cabello F, Garrido F (2007) Role of altered expression of HLA class I molecules in cancer progression. Adv Exp Med Biol 601:123–131

Barnstable CJ, Bodmer WF, Brown G, Galfre G, Milstein C, Williams AF, Ziegler A (1978) Production of monoclonal antibodies to group A erythrocytes, HLA and other human cell surface antigens-new tools for genetic analysis. Cell 14(1):9–20

Benitez R, Godelaine D, Lopez-Nevot MA, Brasseur F, Jiménez P, Marchand M, Oliva MR, van Baren N, Cabrera T, Andry G, Landry C, Ruiz-Cabello F, Boon T, Garrido F (1998) Mutations of the beta2-microglobulin gene result in a lack of HLA class I molecules on melanoma cells of two patients immunized with MAGE peptides. Tissue Antigens 52(6):520–529

Bernal M, Ruiz-Cabello F, Concha A, Paschen A, Garrido F (2012) Implication of the β2-microglobulin gene in the generation of tumor escape phenotypes. Cancer Immunol Immunother 61(9):1359–1371

Blades RA, Keating PJ, McWilliam LJ, George NJ, Stern PL (1995) Loss of HLA class I expression in prostate cancer: implications for immunotherapy. Urology 46(5):681–686

Browning M, Petronzelli F, Bicknell D, Krausa P, Rowan A, Tonks S, Murray N, Bodmer J, Bodmer W (1996) Mechanisms of loss of HLA class I expression on colorectal tumor cells. Tissue Antigens 47(5):364–371

Cabrera CM, Jiménez P, Cabrera T, Esparza C, Ruiz-Cabello F, Garrido F (2003a) Total loss of MHC class I in colorectal tumors can be explained by two molecular pathways: beta2-microglobulin inactivation in MSI-positive tumors and LMP7/TAP2 downregulation in MSI-negative tumors. Tissue Antigens 61(3):211–219

Cabrera CM, López-Nevot MA, Jiménez P, Garrido F (2005) Involvement of the chaperone tapasin in HLA-B44 allelic losses in colorectal tumors. Int J Cancer 113(4):611–618

Cabrera T, Angustias Fernandez M, Sierra A, Garrido A, Herruzo A, Escobedo A, Fabra A, Garrido F (1996) High frequency of altered HLA class I phenotypes in invasive breast carcinomas. Hum Immunol 50(2):127–134

Cabrera T, Collado A, Fernandez MA, Ferron A, Sancho J, Ruiz-Cabello F, Garrido F (1998) High frequency of altered HLA class I phenotypes in invasive colorectal carcinomas. Tissue Antigens 52(2):114–123

Cabrera T, Lara E, Romero JM, Maleno I, Real LM, Ruiz-Cabello F, Valero P, Camacho FM, Garrido F (2007) HLA class I expression in metastatic melanoma correlates with tumor development during autologous vaccination. Cancer Immunol Immunother 56(5):709–717

Cabrera T, López-Nevot MA, Gaforio JJ, Ruiz-Cabello F, Garrido F (2003b) Analysis of HLA expression in human tumor tissues. Cancer Immunol Immunother 52(1):1–9

Cabrera T, Salinero J, Fernandez MA, Garrido A, Esquivias J, Garrido F (2000) High frequency of altered HLA class I phenotypes in laryngeal carcinomas. Hum Immunol 61(5):499–506

Cabrera CM, Jimenez P, Cabrera T, Ruiz-Cabello F, Garrido F (2003c) Molecular mechanisms involved in the total loss of HLA class I in colorectal tumors: 2 m inactivation and LMP7 downregulation. Genes Immun 4:129

Campoli M, Chang CC, Ferrone S (2002) HLA class I antigen loss, tumor immune escape and immune selection. Vaccine 20(Suppl 4):A40–A45

Carosella ED, Moreau P, Le Maoult J, Le Discorde M, Dausset J, Rouas-Freiss N (2003) HLA-G molecules: From maternal-fetal tolerance to tissue acceptance. Adv Immunol 81:199–252

Carretero R, Cabrera T, Gil H, Saenz-Lopez P, Maleno I, Aptsiauri N, Cozar JM, Garrido F (2011) Bacillus Calmette-Guerin immunotherapy of bladder cancer induces selection of human leukocyte antigen class I-deficient tumor cells. Int J Cancer 129(4):839–846

Carretero R, Romero JM, Ruiz-Cabello F, Maleno I, Rodriguez F, Camacho FM, Real LM, Garrido F, Cabrera T (2008) Analysis of HLA class I expression in progressing and regressing metastatic melanoma lesions after immunotherapy. Immunogenetics 60(8):439–447

Carretero R, Wang E, Rodriguez AI, Reinboth J, Ascierto ML, Engle AM, Liu H, Camacho FM, Marincola FM, Garrido F, Cabrera T (2012) Regression of melanoma metastases after immunotherapy is associated with activation of antigen presentation and interferon-mediated rejection genes. Int J Cancer 131(2):387–395

Chang CC, Campoli M, Ferrone S (2003) HLA class I defects in malignant lesions: what have we learned? Keio J Med 52(4):220–229

Chang CC, Campoli M, Ferrone S (2005) Classical and nonclassical HLA class I antigen and NK Cell-activating ligand changes in malignant cells: current challenges and future directions. Adv Cancer Res 93:189–234

Chen HL, Gabrilovich D, Tampé R, Girgis KR, Nadaf S, Carbone DP (1996) A functionally defective allele of TAP1 results in loss of MHC class I antigen presentation in a human lung cancer. Nat Genet 13(2):210–213

Drénou B, Tilanus M, Semana G, Alizadeh M, Birebent B, Grosset JM, Dias P, van Wichen D, Arts Y, De Santis D, Fauchet R, Amiot L (2004) Loss of heterozygosity, a frequent but a non-exclusive mechanism responsible for HLA dysregulation in non-Hodgkin's lymphomas. Br J Haematol 127(1):40–49

Feenstra M, Rozemuller E, Duran K, Stuy I, van den Tweel J, Slootweg P, de Weger R, Tilanus M (1999) Mutation in the beta 2 m gene is not a frequent event in head and neck squamous cell carcinomas. Hum Immunol 60(8):697–706

Feenstra M, Verdaasdonk M, van der Zwan AW, de Weger R, Slootweg P, Tilanus M (2000) Microsatellite analysis of microdissected tumor cells and 6p high density microsatellite analysis in head and neck squamous cell carcinomas with down-regulated human leukocyte antigen class I expression. Lab Invest 80(3):405–414

Garcia-Lora A, Algarra I, Garrido F (2003) MHC class I antigens, immune surveillance, and tumor immune escape. J Cell Physiol 195(3):346–355

Garrido F, Cabrera T, Accolla RS, Bensa JC, Bodmer W, Dohr G, Drouet M, Fauchet R, Ferrara GB, Ferrone S, Giacomini P, Kageshita T, Koopman L, Maio M, Marincola F, Mazzilli C, Morel PA, Murray A, Papasteriades CRH, Salvaneschi L, Stern PL, Ziegler A (1997) HLA and cancer: 12th international histocompatibility workshop study. HLA, Genetic diversity of HLA. Functional and medical implications. vol. I. In: Charron D, EDK (eds). pp 445–452

Garrido F, Cabrera T, Aptsiauri N (2010) "Hard" and "soft" lesions underlying the HLA class I alterations in cancer cells: implications for immunotherapy. Int J Cancer 127(2):249–256

Garrido F, Cabrera T, Concha A, Glew S, Ruiz-Cabello F, Stern PL (1993) Natural history of HLA expression during tumour development. Immunol Today 14(10):491–499

Garrido F, Festenstein H, Schirrmacher V (1976a) Further evidence for depression of H-2 and Ia-like specificities of foreign haplotypes in mouse tumour cell lines. Nature 261(5562):705–707

Garrido F, Ruiz-Cabello F, Cabrera T, Pérez-Villar JJ, López-Botet M, Duggan-Keen M, Stern PL (1997b) Implications for immunosurveillance of altered HLA class I phenotypes in human tumours. Immunol Today 18(2):89–95

Garrido F, Schirrmacher V, Festenstein H (1976b) H-2-like specificities of foreign haplotypes appearing on a mouse sarcoma after vaccinia virus infection. Nature 259(5540):228–230

Hanagiri T, Shigematsu Y, Kuroda K, Baba T, Shiota H, Ichiki Y, Nagata Y, Yasuda M, Uramoto H, So T, Takenoyama M, Tanaka F (2012) Prognostic implications of human leukocyte antigen class I expression in patients who underwent surgical resection for non-small-cell lung cancer. J Surg Res. Jul 31. http://dx.doi.org/10.1016/j.jss.2012.07.029 [Epub ahead of print]

Jiménez P, Cabrera T, Méndez R, Esparza C, Cozar JM, Tallada M, López-Nevot MA, Ruiz-Cabello F, Garrido F (2001) A nucleotide insertion in exon 4 is responsible for the absence of expression of an HLA-A*0301 allele in a prostate carcinoma cell line. Immunogenetics 53(7):606–610

Kageshita T, Ishihara T, Campoli M, Ferrone S (2005) Selective monomorphic and polymorphic HLA class I antigenic determinant loss in surgically removed melanoma lesions. Tissue Antigens 65(5):419–428

Kaneko K, Ishigami S, Kijima Y, Funasako Y, Hirata M, Okumura H, Shinchi H, Koriyama C, Ueno S, Yoshinaka H, Natsugoe S (2011) Clinical implication of HLA class I expression in breast cancer. BMC Cancer 11:454

Kantoff PW, Higano CS, Shore ND, Berger ER, Small EJ, Penson DF, Redfern CH, Ferrari AC, Dreicer R, Sims RB, Xu Y, Frohlich MW, Schellhammer PF, IMPACT Study Investigators (2010) Sipuleucel-T immunotherapy for castration-resistant prostate cancer. N Engl J Med 363(5):411–422

Kikuchi E, Yamazaki K, Torigoe T, Cho Y, Miyamoto M, Oizumi S, Hommura F, Dosaka-Akita H, Nishimura M (2007) HLA class I antigen expression is associated with a favorable prognosis in early stage non-small cell lung cancer. Cancer Sci 98(9):1424–1430

Klebanoff CA, Acquavella N, Yu Z, Restifo NP (2011) Therapeutic cancer vaccines: are we there yet? Immunol Rev 239(1):27–44

Koopman LA, Corver WE, van der Slik AR, Giphart MJ, Fleuren GJ (2000) Multiple genetic alterations cause frequent and heterogeneous human histocompatibility leukocyte antigen class I loss in cervical cancer. J Exp Med 191(6):961–976

Lampen MH, van Hall T (2011) Strategies to counteract MHC-I defects in tumors. Curr Opin Immunol 23(2):293–298

Lehmann F, Marchand M, Hainaut P, Pouillart P, Sastre X, Ikeda H, Boon T, Coulie PG (1995) Differences in the antigens recognized by cytolytic T cells on two successive metastases of a melanoma patient are consistent with immune selection. Eur J Immunol 25(2):340–347

Madjd Z, Spendlove I, Pinder SE, Ellis IO, Durrant LG (2005) Total loss of MHC class I is an independent indicator of good prognosis in breast cancer. Int J Cancer 117(2):248–255

Maleno I, Aptsiauri N, Cabrera T, Gallego A, Paschen A, López-Nevot MA, Garrido F (2011) Frequent loss of heterozygosity in the β2-microglobulin region of chromosome 15 in primary human tumors. Immunogenetics 63(2):65–71

Maleno I, Cabrera CM, Cabrera T, Paco L, López-Nevot MA, Collado A, Ferrón A, Garrido F (2004a) Distribution of HLA class I altered phenotypes in colorectal carcinomas: high frequency of HLA haplotype loss associated with loss of heterozygosity in chromosome region 6p21. Immunogenetics 56(4):244–253

Maleno I, López-Nevot MA, Cabrera T, Salinero J, Garrido F (2002) Multiple mechanisms generate HLA class I altered phenotypes in laryngeal carcinomas: high frequency of HLA haplotype loss associated with loss of heterozygosity in chromosome region 6p21. Cancer Immunol Immunother 51(7):389–396

Maleno I, Romero JM, Cabrera T, Paco L, Aptsiauri N, Cozar JM, Tallada M, López-Nevot MA, Garrido F (2006) LOH at 6p21.3 region and HLA class I altered phenotypes in bladder carcinomas. Immunogenetics 58(7):503–510

Marincola FM, Jaffee EM, Hicklin DJ, Ferrone S (2000) Escape of human solid tumors from T-cell recognition: molecular mechanisms and functional significance. Adv Immunol 74: 181–273

Martini M, Testi MG, Pasetto M, Picchio MC, Innamorati G, Mazzocco M, Ugel S, Cingarlini S, Bronte V, Zanovello P, Krampera M, Mosna F, Cestari T, Riviera AP, Brutti N, Barbieri O, Matera L, Tridente G, Colombatti M, Sartoris S (2010) IFN-gamma-mediated upmodulation of MHC class I expression activates tumor-specific immune response in a mouse model of prostate cancer. Vaccine 28(20):3548–3557

Meissner M, Reichert TE, Kunkel M, Gooding W, Whiteside TL, Ferrone S, Seliger B (2005) Defects in the human leukocyte antigen class I antigen-processing machinery in head and neck squamous cell carcinoma: Association with clinical outcome. Clin Cancer Res 11(7): 2552–2560

Menon AG, Morreau H, Tollenaar RA, Alphenaar E, Van Puijenbroek M, Putter H, Janssen-Van Rhijn CM, Van De Velde CJ, Fleuren GJ, Kuppen PJ (2002) Down-regulation of HLA-A expression correlates with a better prognosis in colorectal cancer patients. Lab Invest 82(12):1725–1733

Miyagi T, Tatsumi T, Takehara T, Kanto T, Kuzushita N, Sugimoto Y, Jinushi M, Kasahara A, Sasaki Y, Hori M, Hayashi N (2003) Impaired expression of proteasome subunits and human leukocyte antigens class I in human colon cancer cells. J Gastroenterol Hepatol 18(1):32–40

Morabito A, Dozin B, Salvi S, Pasciucco G, Balbi G, Laurent S, Pastorino S, Carli F, Truini M, Bruzzi P, Del Mastro L, Pistillo MP (2009) Analysis and clinical relevance of human leukocyte antigen class I, heavy chain, and beta2-microglobulin downregulation in breast cancer. Hum Immunol 70(7):492–495

Paschen A, Arens N, Sucker A, Greulich-Bode KM, Fonsatti E, Gloghini A, Striegel S, Schwinn N, Carbone A, Hildenbrand R, Cerwenka A, Maio M, Schadendorf D (2006) The coincidence of chromosome 15 aberrations and beta2-microglobulin gene mutations is causative for the total loss of human leukocyte antigen class I expression in melanoma. Clin Cancer Res 12(11 Pt 1):3297–3305

Paschen A, Méndez RM, Jimenez P, Sucker A, Ruiz-Cabello F, Song M, Garrido F, Schadendorf D (2003) Complete loss of HLA class I antigen expression on melanoma cells: a result of successive mutational events. Int J Cancer 103(6):759–767

Pérez B, Benitez R, Fernández MA, Oliva MR, Soto JL, Serrano S, López Nevot MA, Garrido F (1999) A new beta 2 microglobulin mutation found in a melanoma tumor cell line. Tissue Antigens 53(6):569–572

Ploegh HL (1998) Viral strategies of immune evasion. Science 280(5361):248–253

Powell AG, Horgan PG, Edwards J (2012) The bodies fight against cancer: is human leukocyte antigen (HLA) class 1 the key? J Cancer Res Clin Oncol 138(5):723–728

Ramnath N, Tan D, Li Q, Hylander BL, Bogner P, Ryes L, Ferrone S (2006) Is downregulation of MHC class I antigen expression in human non-small cell lung cancer associated with prolonged survival? Cancer Immunol Immunother 55(8):891–899

Restifo NP, Marincola FM, Kawakami Y, Taubenberger J, Yannelli JR, Rosenberg SA (1996) Loss of functional beta(2)-microglobulin in metastatic melanomas from five patients receiving immunotherapy. J Natl Cancer Inst 88(2):100–108

Rodriguez T, Mendez R, Del Campo A, Jimenez P, Aptsiauri N, Garrido F, Ruiz-Cabello F (2007) Distinct mechanisms of loss of IFN-gamma mediated HLA class I inducibility in two melanoma cell lines. BMC Cancer 7:34

Rodriguez T, Méndez R, Roberts CH, Ruiz-Cabello F, Dodi IA, López Nevot MA, Paco L, Maleno I, Marsh SG, Pawelec G, Garrido F (2005) High frequency of homozygosity of the HLA region in melanoma cell lines reveals a pattern compatible with extensive loss of heterozygosity. Cancer Immunol Immunother 54(2):141–148

Rosenberg SA, Yang JC, Restifo NP (2004) Cancer immunotherapy: moving beyond current vaccines. Nat Med 10(9):909–915

Ryschich E, Cebotari O, Fabian OV, Autschbach F, Kleeff J, Friess H, Bierhaus A, Büchler MW, Schmidt J (2004) Loss of heterozygosity in the HLA class I region in human pancreatic cancer. Tissue Antigens 64(6):696–702

Schlom J (2012) Recent advances in therapeutic cancer vaccines. Cancer Biother Radiopharm 27(1):2–5

Seliger B, Maeurer MJ, Ferrone S (2000) Antigen-processing machinery breakdown and tumor growth. Immunol Today 21(9):455–464

Seliger B, Ritz U, Abele R, Bock M, Tampé R, Sutter G, Drexler I, Huber C, Ferrone S (2001) Immune escape of melanoma: first evidence of structural alterations in two distinct components of the MHC class I antigen processing pathway. Cancer Res 61(24):8647–8650

Seliger B, Ruiz-Cabello F, Garrido F (2008) IFN inducibility of major histocompatibility antigens in tumors. Adv Cancer Res 101:249–276

Serrano A, Brady CS, Jimenez P, Duggan-Keen MF, Mendez R, Stern P, Garrido F, Ruiz-Cabello F (2000) A mutation determining the loss of HLA-A2 antigen expression in a cervical carcinoma reveals novel splicing of human MHC class I classical transcripts in both tumoral and normal cells. Immunogenetics 51(12):1047–1052

Serrano A, Tanzarella S, Lionello I, Mendez R, Traversari C, Ruiz-Cabello F, Garrido F (2001) Rexpression of HLA class I antigens and restoration of antigen-specific CTL response in melanoma cells following 5-aza-2'-deoxycytidine treatment. Int J Cancer 94(2):243–251

Speetjens FM, de Bruin EC, Morreau H, Zeestraten EC, Putter H, van Krieken JH, van Buren MM, van Velzen M, Dekker-Ensink NG, van de Velde CJ, Kuppen PJ (2008) Clinical impact of HLA class I expression in rectal cancer. Cancer Immunol Immunother 57(5):601–609

Torres MJ, Ruiz-Cabello F, Skoudy A, Berrozpe G, Jimenez P, Serrano A, Real FX, Garrido F (1996) Loss of an HLA haplotype in pancreas cancer tissue and its corresponding tumor derived cell line. Tissue Antigens 47(5):372–381

van der Bruggen P, Traversari C, Chomez P, Lurquin C, De Plaen E, Van den Eynde B, Knuth A, Boon T (1991) A gene encoding an antigen recognized by cytolytic T lymphocytes on a human melanoma. Science 254(5038):1643–1647

Walter S, Weinschenk T, Stenzl A, Zdrojowy R, Pluzanska A, Szczylik C, Staehler M, Brugger W, Dietrich PY, Mendrzyk R, Hilf N, Schoor O, Fritsche J, Mahr A, Maurer D, Vass V, Trautwein C, Lewandrowski P, Flohr C, Pohla H, Stanczak JJ, Bronte V, Mandruz-zato S, Biedermann T, Pawelec G, Derhovanessian E, Yamagishi H, Miki T, Hongo F, Takaha N, Hirakawa K, Tanaka H, Stevanovic S, Frisch J, Mayer-Mokler A, Kirner A, Rammensee HG, Reinhardt C, Singh-Jasuja H. Multipeptide immune response to cancer vaccine IMA901 after single-dose cyclophosphamide associates with longer pa-tient survival. Nat Med. 2012 Jul 29. doi: 10.1038/nm.2883. [Epub ahead of print]

Watson NF, Ramage JM, Madjd Z, Spendlove I, Ellis IO, Scholefield JH, Durrant LG (2006) Immunosurveillance is active in colorectal cancer as downregulation but not complete loss of MHC class I expression correlates with a poor prognosis. Int J Cancer 118(1):6–10

Yoon SJ, Kang JO, Park JS, Kim NK, Heo DS (2000) Reduced expression of MHC class I antigen in human cancer cell lines with defective LMP-7. Anticancer Res 20(2A):949–953

Chapter 3
MHC Class I Expression in Experimental Mouse Models of Cancer: Immunotherapy of Tumors with Different MHC-I Expression Patterns

In this chapter, we analyze the role of tumor MHC-I cell surface expression in the success of various types of cancer immunotherapy in several mouse models of cancer. First, we show how different immunotherapies influence the growth of MHC-I-positive or -deficient primary tumors. We also describe how MHC-I expression on primary tumors determine the success of immunotherapy in control of metastatic progression. Finally, we support the role of tumor MHC-I cell surface expression in success of immunotherapy against metastatic disease, by describing our recent results obtained from a murine fibrosarcoma model, a heterogeneous tumor composed of various tumor cell clones with different MHC-I expression. We performed spontaneous metastasis assays with different cell clones derived from a primary fibrosarcoma tumor induced by methylcholanthrene (MCA) in BALB/c mice. These fibrosarcoma clones have distinct patterns of MHC-I cell surface expression, ranging from MHC-I-negative to MHC-I-highly positive expression. Each clone has different spontaneous metastatic capacity, which correlates directly with its MHC-I cell surface expression. Clones with high MHC-I expression demonstrated high spontaneous metastatic capacity. Two types of immunotherapy, chemotherapy alone, and chemoimmunotherapy, were applied separately to treat spontaneous metastatic colonization generated by the different fibrosarcoma clones. The results showed that the success of the immunotherapy against metastatic disease depends on MHC-I cell surface expression on fibrosarcoma cells. Spontaneous metastatic capacity presented by a highly positive MHC-I fibrosarcoma clone was completely abrogated by immunotherapies and chemo-immunotherapy. In contrast, metastatic disease derived from a fibrosarcoma clone with intermediate MHC-I levels was only partially inhibited. These results indicate that MHC-I cell surface expression in primary tumor may be crucial for the success of immunotherapy against metastatic disease.

N. Aptsiauri et al., *MHC Class I Antigens In Malignant Cells: Immune Escape and Response to Immunotherapy*, SpringerBriefs in Cancer Research 6, DOI 10.1007/978-1-4614-6543-0_3, © Teresa Cabrera 2013

Immunotherapy of Primary Tumors with Different Levels of MHC-I Expression

The correlation between the efficacy of immunotherapy to inhibit primary tumor progression and the tumor MHC-I cell surface expression has been studied in different murine tumor models. MHC-I cell surface expression level on tumor cells is crucial for the outcome of immunotherapies based on vaccination with peptides derived from tumor associated antigens (TAA). Tumor cells with high expression levels of MHC-I and of tumor antigen are expected to demonstrate a good response to therapy. Loss of MHC-I expression or of a specific tumor antigen might lead to the failure of the treatment. Therefore, it is important to emphasize that before administration of a peptide-based cancer vaccine, tumor cell surface expression of MHC-I molecules and of the specific TAA must be evaluated. Furthermore, it has been recently reported that IFN-γ limits the effectiveness of melanoma peptide vaccines because tumor cells exposed to IFN-γ evade CTLs by inducing large amounts of noncognate MHC-I molecules, which prevent T-cell activation and effector function (Cho et al. 2011). The identification of these noncognate MHC-I molecules and conditions in which they are induced, as well as a correlation with the MHC-I classical expression on tumor cells, seems to be important for the improvement of the success of vaccination with peptides. Recently, it has been reported that tumor-infiltrating myeloid cells (MDSCs) induce tumor cell resistance to CTLs in mice (Lu et al. 2011). MDSCs segregates the free radical peroxynitrite (PNT), which inhibited binding of processed peptides to MHC-I molecules expressed on tumor cells. These last two immunosuppressive mechanisms show as presentation of TAAs by MHC-I molecules may be inhibited in case when MHC-I cell surface expression and TAA expression is not specifically down-regulated.

In another murine tumor model, B16 melanoma, intratumoral electroporation of IL-12 cDNA used in MHC-I negative tumor cells, produced eradication of established melanomas (Sin et al. 2012). The antitumor effect required the participation of IFN-γ, which upregulated tumor MHC-I expression and increased anti-tumor activity of the specific CD8+ CTLs. Treatment of cervical carcinoma cells with synthetic oligodeoxynucleotide bearing CpG motifs (CpG-ODNs) caused tumor regression, which correlated with MHC-I upregulation (Baines and Celis 2003). The antitumor effect was associated with CD8+ T-cell activation. In contrast, other studies show that CpG-ODNs immunotherapy significantly reduces the growth of both MHC-I-positive and -deficient tumors (Reinis et al. 2006). CpG ODN 1585, whose mechanism of action principally involves activation of NK cells, induced regression only of MHC-I-deficient tumors. Combination of CpG with dendritic cell-based vaccines or vaccination with longer peptides resulted in tumor growth inhibition of both MHC-I-positive and -negative tumors (Reinis et al. 2010). Moreover, CpG-ODNs were equally effective in treatment of minimal residual tumor disease with MHC-I-positive and -negative tumors in a murine model after chemotherapy or surgery (Reinis et al. 2007). In these assays, NK1.1+ cells seem to be important for the development of protective immunity against MHC-I-deficient tumors (Indrova et al. 2011). Furthermore, depletion of T(reg) cells inhibited growth of recurrent tumors after surgery of MHC-I-positive and -deficient tumors transplanted in syngeneic mice (Simova et al. 2006).

Other strategy for the treatment of MHC-I deficient tumors by immunotherapy could be upregulation of tumor cell surface MHC-I expression before the treatment. Frequently, MHC-I down-regulation or antigen silencing is caused by epigenetic mechanisms. In that case treatment with 5-azacytidine (5AC) or with histone deacetylase inhibitor Trichostatin A may increase tumor MHC-I/antigen expression (Manning et al. 2008; Setiadi et al. 2008; Bao et al. 2011). Simova et al. have reported an additive therapeutic effect of a combination of 5AC with CpG-ODN or with IL-12 producing cellular vaccine, in both MHC+ and MHC− tumors (Simova et al. 2011). The efficacy of the combined chemo-immunotherapy against originally MHC class I-deficient tumors was partially dependent on the CD8(+)-mediated immune responses. Increased cell surface expression of MHC class I cell molecules, associated with upregulation of the antigen-presenting machinery-related genes, as well as of genes encoding selected components of the IFNγ-signalling pathway in tumors explanted from 5AC-treated animals, were observed. Chemo-immunotherapy with ifosfamide derivative CBM-4A together with IL-12 also produced a significant inhibition of growth of both MHC-I-deficient and -positive tumors (Indrova et al. 2006).

Immunotherapy Against Metastases Derived from Primary Tumors with Different MHC-I Cell Surface Expression

We considered that only murine spontaneous metastasis assays may reflect really the metastatic progression in humans (Ellis and Fidler 2010). In these assays, to get closer to the cancer treatment protocol in humans, a primary tumor is surgically removed and metastatic cells spread via blood circulation and colonize distant organs. In murine experimental metastasis assays tumor cells are injected directly into the tail vein; this way the first steps of treatment are skipped and metastatic progression does not completely emulate metastatic colonization that takes place in humans. Moreover, immunotherapy as anti-metastatic treatment in murine tumor models should be administered after the removal of the primary tumor, like in cancer patients. Here, we summarize the studies in mice analyzing the relation between the success of immunotherapy as anti-metastatic treatment against spontaneous metastases and MHC-I cell surface expression on primary tumor cells.

Between the 1980s and 1990s, the studies performed by Eisenbach's research group reported an indirect correlation between H 2K tumor cell surface expression and spontaneous metastatic capacity (Eisenbach et al. 1984; Porgador et al. 1991; Feldman and Eisenbach 1991; VandenDriessche et al. 1994a). Tumor cells clones derived from H-2-K-low or -negative tumors, including 3-Lewis lung carcinoma, B16 melanoma, or BW T lymphoma, have increased spontaneous metastatic capacity. Moreover, recovery of the H-2 K expression reverted their metastatic phenotype (Porgador et al. 1993; Mandelboim et al. 1992; Plaksin et al. 1988; VandenDriessche et al. 1994b). Furthermore, injection of the H-2-tranfected cells was successful in eradicating metastases derived from primary tumor originated from parental cells. Therapy with IFN-γ-treated tumor cells or with tumor cells transfected with IFN-γ gene, both promoted induction of MHC-I cell surface expression, and protected against metastatic progression of the parental tumor (Porgador et al. 1991, 1993). If the tumor cells are transfected jointly with IFN-γ and allogeneic MHC class I cDNAs a greater anti-metastatic effect was achieved (Lim et al. 1998).

In our laboratory, we have developed a fibrosarcoma murine model with various cancer cell clones derived from the same primary tumor. These clones are characterized with different MHC-I expression patterns and distinct spontaneous metastatic capacity. Using this model, we observed that high tumor cell surface MHC-I expression correlates with higher spontaneous metastatic capacity and slower local tumor growth (Garrido et al. 1986a, b; Perez et al. 1990; Algarra et al. 1991). We believe that this murine fibrosarcoma model could be a good candidate to elucidate the role of MHC-I expression in the outcome of anti-metastatic immunotherapy. We hypothesize that the clones with high spontaneous metastatic capacity might respond to immunotherapy, since they have high MHC-I expression. In the next section we describe the assays performed and the results found.

Immunotherapy Used as Anti-metastatic Treatment in a Murine Tumor Model Composed of Several Clones with Different MHC-I Expression

GR9 Murine Tumor Model

GR9 murine tumor model was created in our laboratory in the middle of 1980s. BALB/c mice were treated with 3-methylcholanthrene obtaining a fibrosarcoma local tumor (Garrido et al. 1986a). This local tumor was excised and adapted to tissue culture. The tumor cell line obtained was named GR9, and cloned by limit dilution obtaining several clones corresponding to the different tumor cells present in primary tumor GR9. All obtained clones were analyzed for MHC-I surface expression and some of these clones were selected based on different MHC-I phenotypes. GR9 fibrosarcoma cells present intermediate levels of H-2 K^d, D^d and L^d molecules (Fig. 3.1). The G2 and A7 fibrosarcoma clones present high MHC-I cell surface expression, whereas the B7 and C5 clones show MHC-I intermediate levels, and the B11 and B9 fibrosarcoma clones present weak or negative MHC-I cell surface expression (Fig. 3.1). These six clones represent the different MHC-I phenotypes found in GR9 primary tumors.

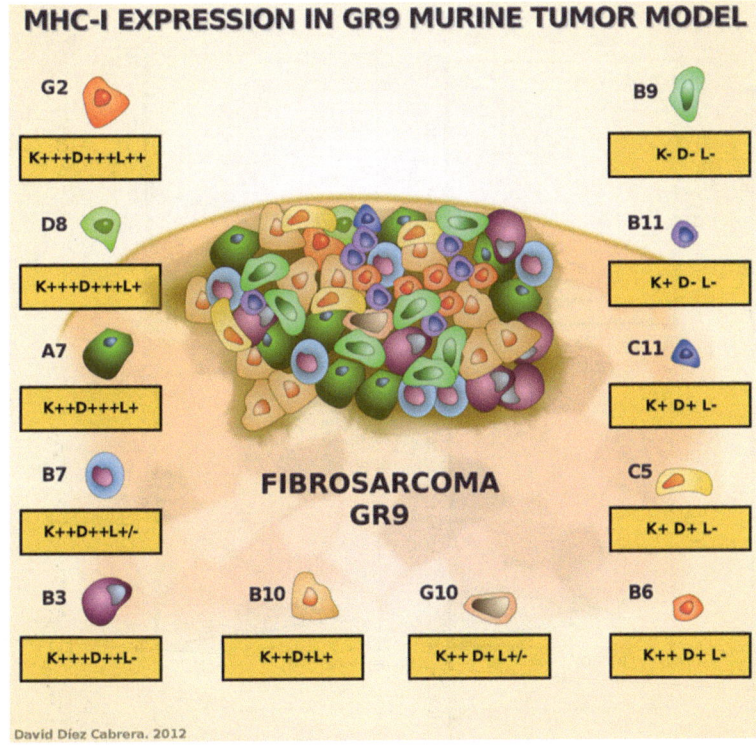

MHC-I EXPRESSION IN GR9 MURINE TUMOR MODEL

G2 — K+++D+++L++

B9 — K- D- L-

D8 — K+++D+++L+

B11 — K+ D- L-

A7 — K++D+++L+

C11 — K+ D+ L-

B7 — K++D++L+/-

C5 — K+ D+ L-

FIBROSARCOMA GR9

B3 — K+++D++L-

B10 — K++D+L+

G10 — K++ D+ L+/-

B6 — K++ D+ L-

David Díez Cabrera. 2012

Fig. 3.1 All clones adapted to tissue culture from the primary tumor GR9. The clones are depicted according to MHC-I cell surface expression (H-2 K^d, D^d and L^d molecules)

Four clones, representing all MHC-I phenotypes found, were selected for the studies: A7, B7, C5, and B11. Figure 3.2 depicts quantitative MHC-I cell surface expression measured by flow cytometry of these four clones. The MHC-I expression range from highly positive A7 clone to weakly positive B11 clone, which expresses only a low level of H-2 K molecule. In all cases, the three H-2 molecules are induced after IFN-γ treatment (Fig. 3.2). This last result indicates that down-regulation of MHC-I expression in these clones is due to reversible MHC-I alterations, "soft lesions."

In Vivo Local Growth and Metastatic Capacity of the Studied Fibrosarcoma Clones

Several cell doses of each fibrosarcoma clones were injected subcutaneously in BALB/c mice and the results depicted an indirect correlation between MHC-I surface expression and local tumor growth rate. The clone with lower level of MHC-I expression, B11, showed higher local growth rate, followed by C5, and finally B7

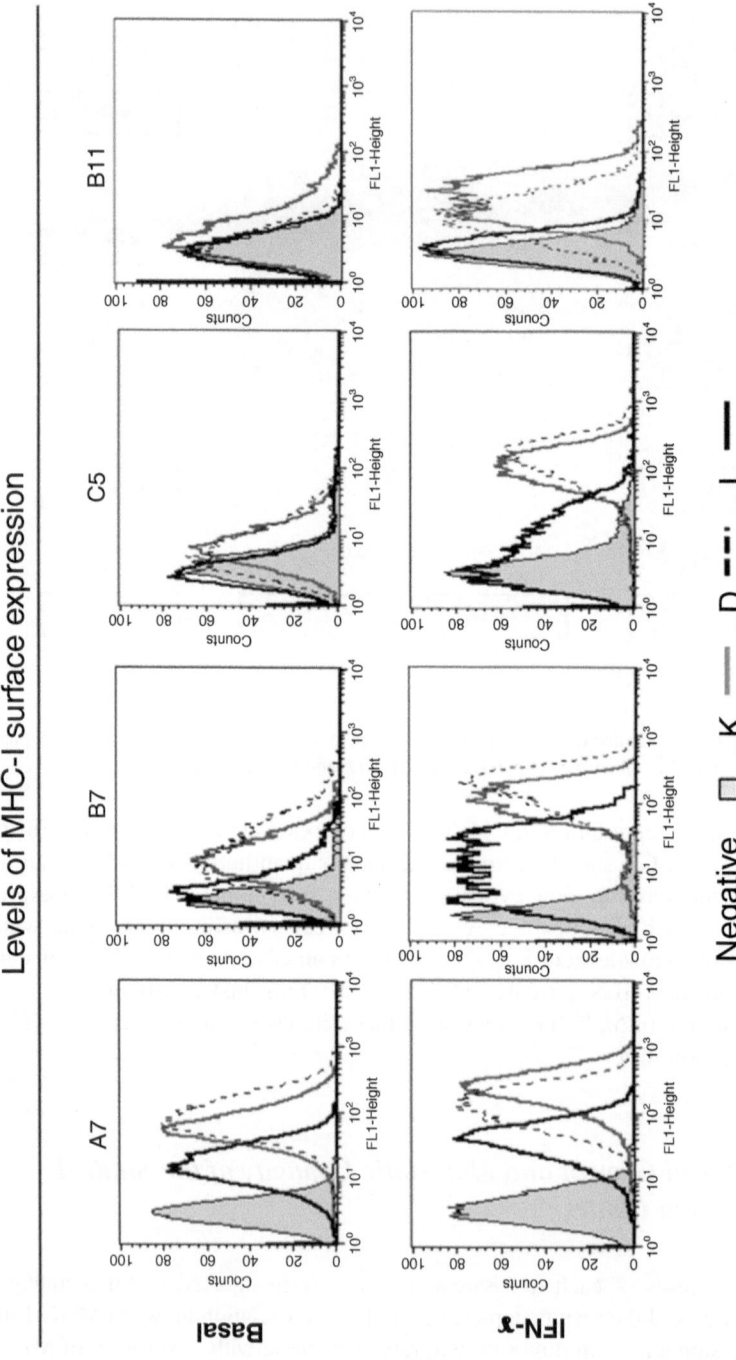

Fig. 3.2 MHC-I cell surface expression in four clones of GR9 fibrosarcoma. Flow cytometry assays measuring MHC-I cell surface expression on four different clones derived from GR9 tumor

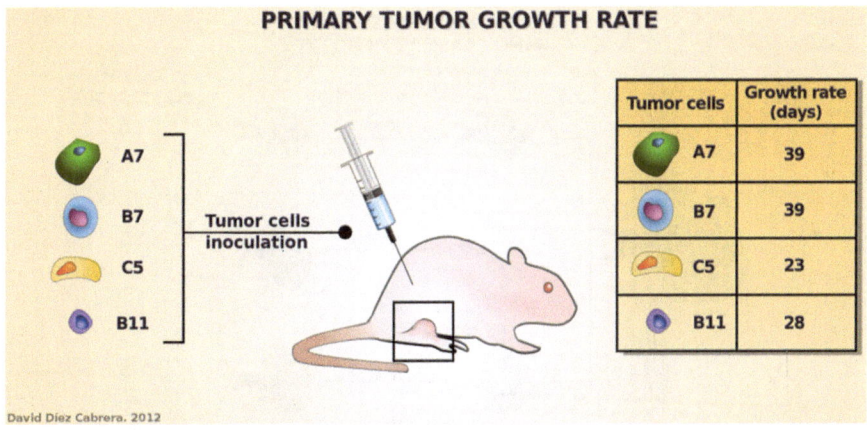

Fig. 3.3 Local tumor growth rate of the four different clones of GR9 fibrosarcoma model. C5 and B11 clones presented higher growth rate than A7 and B7 clones

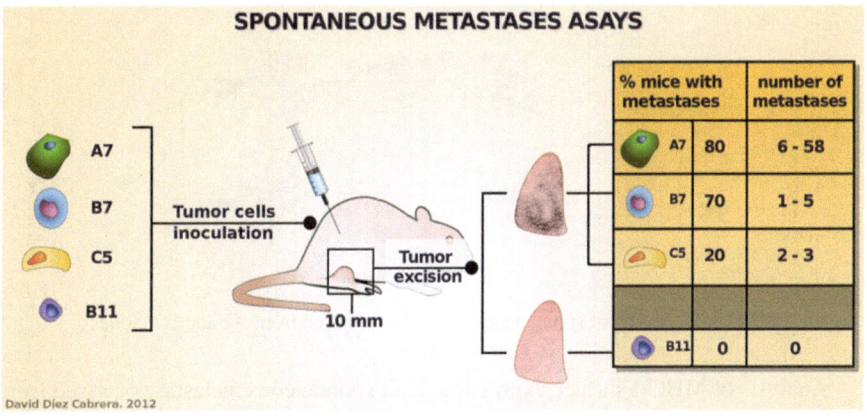

Fig. 3.4 Spontaneous metastatic capacity of four clones of GR9 tumor. A7 clone presented a high metastatic capacity, whereas than B7 and C5 clones presented a weak metastatic capacity. B11 clone did not produce metastases

and A7 clones (Fig. 3.3). Thus, B11 and C5 clones presented higher growth rate than A7 and B7 clones.

In spontaneous metastasis assays we obtained opposite results, showing a direct correlation between MHC-I phenotype and spontaneous metastatic capacity of the fibrosarcoma clones (Fig. 3.4). The MHC-I more positive clone A7 presented highest spontaneous metastatic capacity, whereas that B7 and C5 clones showed a weak spontaneous metastatic capacity, while B11 did not generate spontaneous metastases for any of the injected doses. GR9 fibrosarcoma cells presented high metastatic capacity.

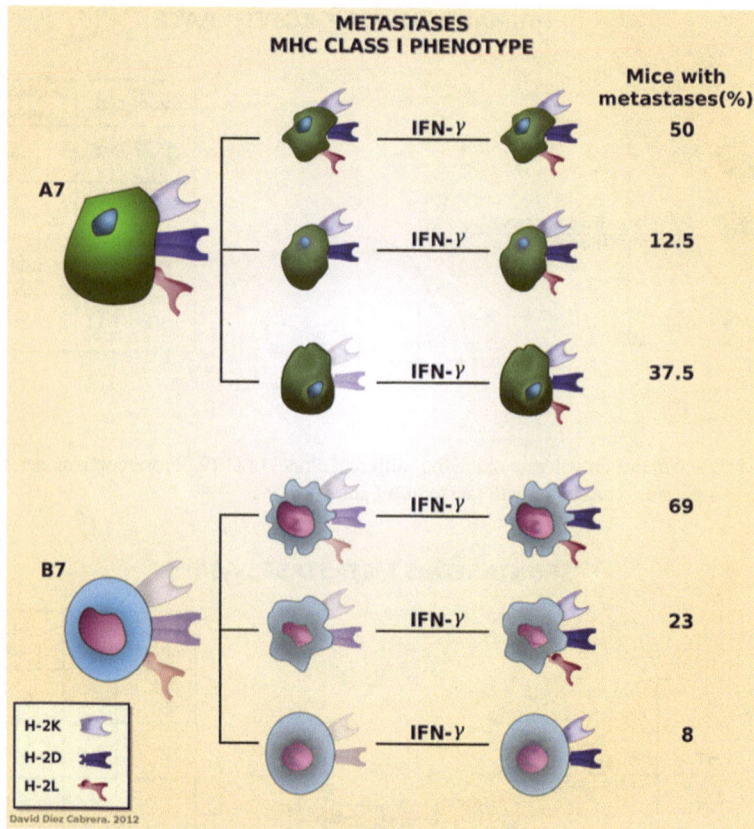

Fig. 3.5 MHC-I phenotype of spontaneous metastases derived from A7 and B7 clones

Analysis of MHC-I surface expression in all spontaneous metastases derived from different fibrosarcoma clones or from GR9 cells, showed that in all cases the spontaneous metastases presented the same or lower MHC-I surface expression than the clone from which they were originated. All metastases generated from A7 clone had reversible MHC-I alterations, "soft lesions," recovering MHC-I cell surface expression after IFN treatment (Garrido et al. 2011). In contrast, metastases derived from B7 clone had soft MHC-I lesions or structural alterations, "hard lesions" (Fig. 3.5).

Immunotherapy as Anti-metastatic Treatment of A7 Fibrosarcoma Clone with High Level of MHC-I Expression

A7 is a highly MHC-I-positive clone with strong spontaneous metastatic capacity (5–50 metastases per animal). Two types of immunotherapy, one chemotherapy and one chemo-immunotherapy protocols were administered to BALB/c mice injected

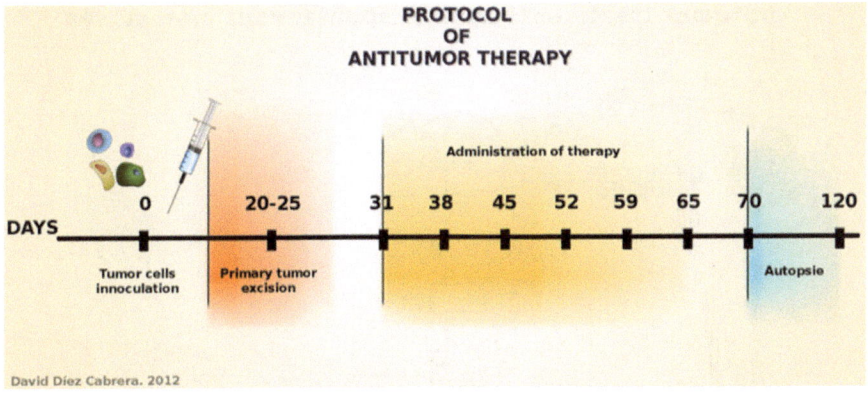

Fig. 3.6 Time course of treatment protocols. Therapies were administered as weekly intraperitoneal injections for 6 weeks, beginning 1 week after removal of the primary tumor. Ten mice were euthanized on day 70 to analyze treatment efficacy. Remaining 10 mice were sacrificed on day 120 to evaluate the long-term effect. In control and docetaxel group all mice were sacrificed on day 70

with A7 tumor cells or to wild type BALB/c mice to evaluate their anti-metastatic capacity (Garrido et al. 2011). Protein bound polysaccharide K (PSK) (Fisher and Yang 2002), and CpG+ irradiated autologous A7 tumor cells were used as immunotherapy treatments, docetaxel as chemotherapy, and PSK+ docetaxel as chemoimmunotherapy. A7 tumor cells were injected subcutaneously and when the large tumor diameter reached 10 mm, the primary tumor was removed. One week after the excision of the primary tumor, the treatments began on a weekly basis during 6 weeks. One week after the last dose, mice were euthanized and autopsy was performed (Fig. 3.6).

Surprisingly, all mice treated with immunotherapy or chemo-immunotherapy did not develop any metastases (Fig. 3.7). In other assays, the mice were free of metastasis for up to 6 months after the administration of the last dose of treatment. Chemotherapy treatment promoted a partial reduction in the number of metastases. The control group, mice injected with A7 cells and treated with saline, developed a high number of spontaneous metastases. These results indicate that the two immunotherapy protocols and the chemo-immunotherapy protocol eradicated completely metastatic colonization and cured the mice, whereas that chemotherapy protocol only reduced the number of metastases (Fig. 3.7).

Analysis of lymphocyte subpopulations, comparing wild type mice with mice injected with A7 fibrosarcoma cells, showed that growth of A7 primary tumor promote the immunosuppression of the host (Fig. 3.8) (Garrido et al. 2011). Treg cells were increased, and T-CD4+ lymphocyte and T-CD8+ lymphocyte subpopulations decreased in the injected mice. Application of the two immunotherapies and one chemo-immunotherapy reverted this immunosuppression, even promoting an immunostimulation that directly correlated with the anti-metastatic effects observed.

In brief, the results show that immunotherapy treatments were successful against spontaneous metastatic colonization generated from A7 fibrosarcoma clone.

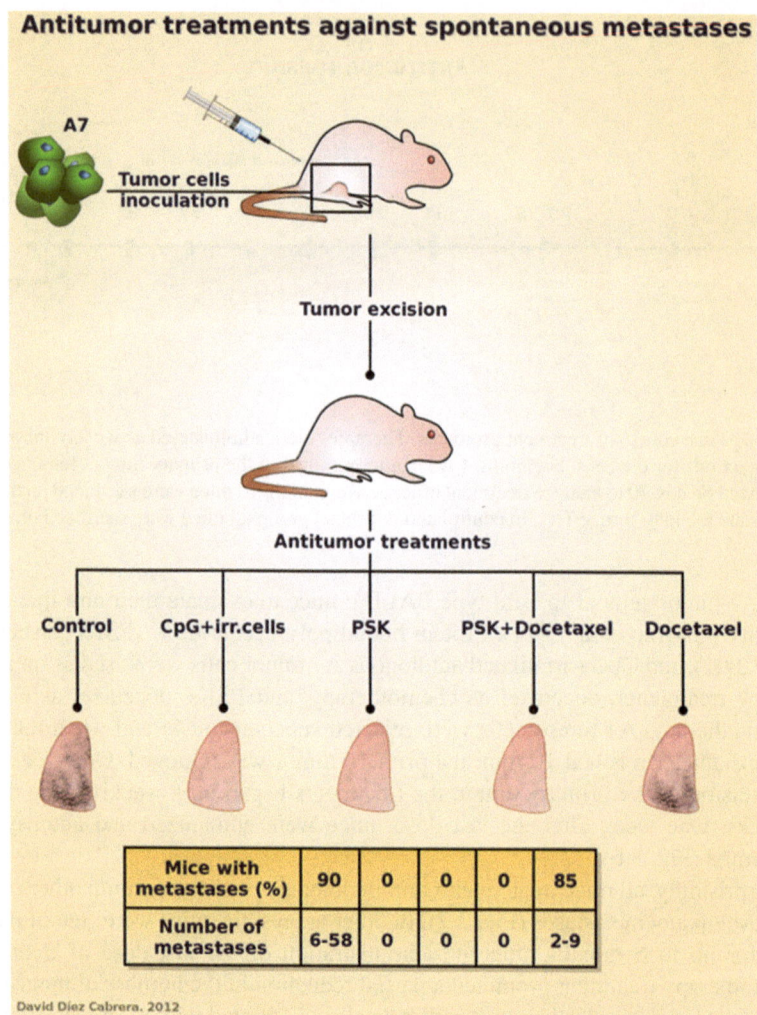

Fig. 3.7 Spontaneous metastases in A7-injected mice treated with different therapies. At the end of treatment mice were euthanized (day 70 and 120 post-cell injection). The figure depicts % of mice with metastases and number of pulmonary metastases (PM) per mouse. The two immunotherapies and the chemo-immunotherapy eradicated metastases. However, chemotherapy alone only reduced the number of metastases

Immunotherapy as Anti-metastatic Treatment of B7 Clone with an Intermediate Level of MHC-I Expression

Previously described immunotherapy, chemotherapy or chemo-immunotherapy were also applied for metastatic colonization generated from B7 fibrosarcoma clone, which has an intermediate MHC-I expression level (Fig. 3.1). In this case, the

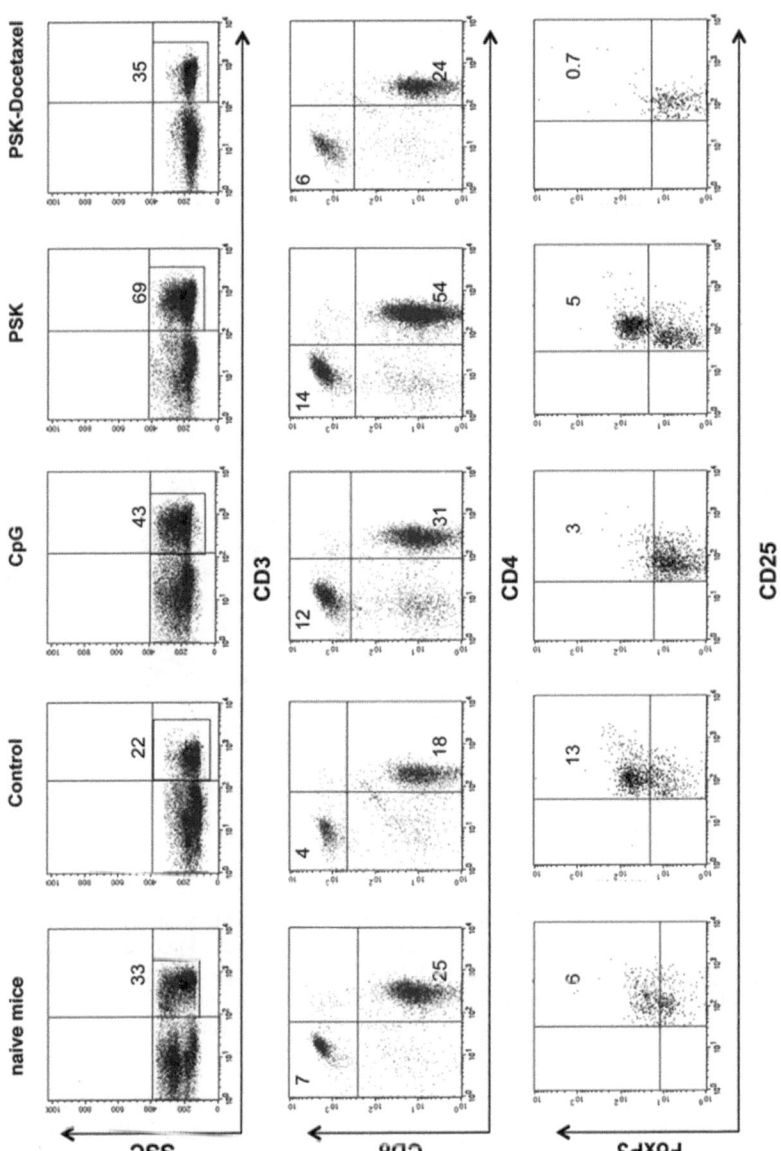

Fig. 3.8 Spleen lymphocyte subpopulations (%) were analyzed in naive mice and in mice from control and immunotherapy groups. A representative experiment determining T lymphocytes subpopulations (CD3+ CD4+ and CD3+ CD8+) and Treg cells (CD4+ CD25+ FoxP3+) is depicted. All percentages are referred to total number of lymphocytes except for Treg that is referred to CD4+ cells. Increase in T lymphocyte subpopulations and decrease in Treg cells is observed after of immunotherapy or chemo-immunotherapy treatments

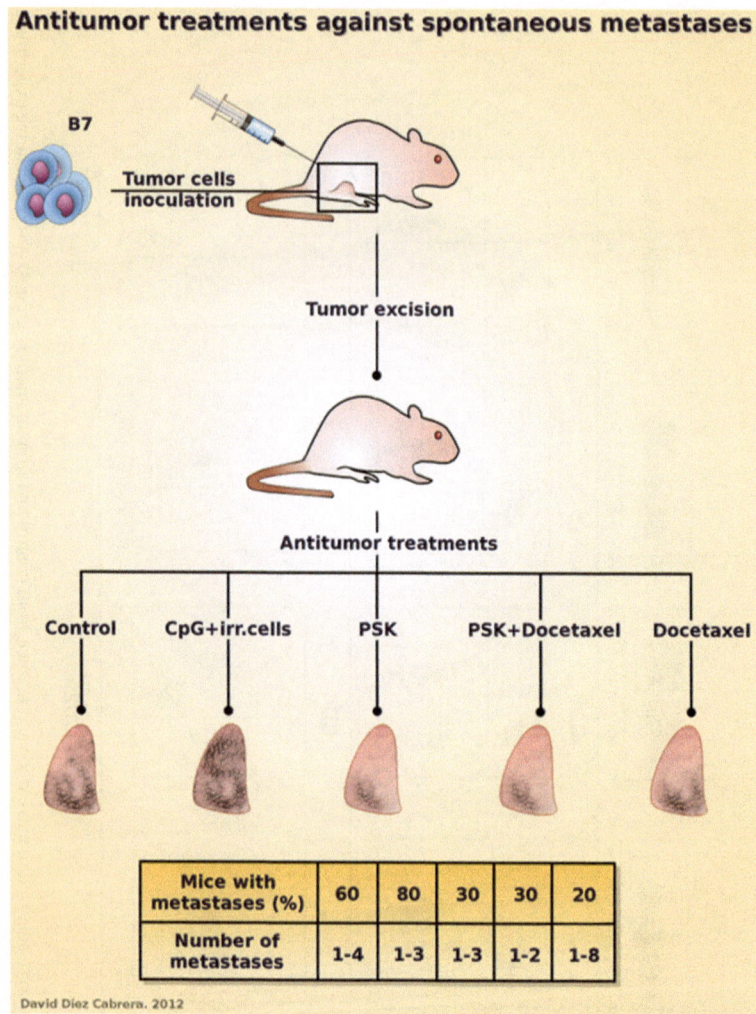

Fig. 3.9 Spontaneous metastases in B7-injected mice treated with different therapies. At the end of treatment mice were euthanized (day 70 and 120 post-cell injection). The figure depicts % of mice with metastases and number of pulmonary metastases (PM) per mouse. The PSK immunotherapy and the chemo-immunotherapy reduced the number of mice with metastases. However, treatment with CpG+ irradiated cells increased the number of mice with metastases

treatments were not as effective as for highly MHC-I positive A7 fibrosarcoma clone (Fig. 3.9). Administration of CpG+ autologous irradiated tumor cells in mice injected with B7 fibrosarcoma clone showed no anti-metastatic effect. Furthermore, the number of animals with metastases were higher with this immunotherapy. The PSK and PSK+ docetaxel treatments reached a partial anti-metastatic activity, reduced the number of mice with metastases and the number of metastases per animal. Docetaxel chemotherapy obtain partial anti-metastatic effect, showing similar metastatic colonization grade than in the PSK group (manuscript in preparation). In brief, PSK immunotherapy and chemo-immunotherapy treatments reached a partial inhibition of metastatic colonization.

Immunotherapy as Anti-metastatic Treatment Against Metastatic Colonization Generated from GR9 Fibrosarcoma Cells

Finally, we applied the same anti-metastatic treatments in mice injected with the original GR9 fibrosarcoma cell line. In this case, all administered treatments were ineffective, and all mice treated showed the same metastatic colonization grade than in control group (unpublished observations).

Chapter Summary

In summary, in GR9 murine tumor model, we have been able to demonstrate to direct relation between successful immunotherapy as anti-metastatic treatment and MHC-I cell surface expression on primary tumor cells. Two immunotherapy treatments were completely effective eradicating metastatic colonization derived from a high MHC-I positive fibrosarcoma clone, which had a high spontaneous metastatic capacity in non-treated mice. Both immunotherapy treatments administered after primary tumor excision reached to maintain the animals free of metastases, eradicating the metastasis spread from A7 tumor clone. Growth of primary tumor promoted a strong immunosuppression, which could be reverted by the immunotherapy treatments. In contrast, the same immunotherapy treatments only produced partial metastatic inhibition when they were administered to the mice carrying primary tumor originated from a B7 fibrosarcoma clone with intermediate MHC-I expression level. This clone also promoted a strong immunosuppression, which only could be reverted partially by immunotherapy treatments. These results indicate that the success of immunotherapy as anti-metastatic treatment may depend strongly of the MHC-I expression level on primary tumor cells. A MHC-I expression threshold on primary tumor cells is necessary so that immunotherapy can be effective against metastatic disease.

References

Algarra I, Gaforio JJ, Garrido A, Mialdea MJ, Perez M, Garrido F (1991) Heterogeneity of MHC-class-I antigens in clones of methylcholanthrene-induced tumors. Implications for local growth and metastasis. Int J Cancer Suppl 6:73–81

Baines J, Celis E (2003) Immune-mediated tumor regression induced by CpG-containing oligodeoxynucleotides. Clin Cancer Res 9(7):2693–2700

Bao L, Dunham K, Lucas K (2011) MAGE-A1, MAGE-A3, and NY-ESO-1 can be upregulated on neuroblastoma cells to facilitate cytotoxic T lymphocyte-mediated tumor cell killing. Cancer Immunol Immunother 60(9):1299–1307

Cho HI, Lee YR, Celis E (2011) Interferon gamma limits the effectiveness of melanoma peptide vaccines. Blood 117(1):135–144

Eisenbach L, Hollander N, Greenfeld L, Yakor H, Segal S, Feldman M (1984) The differential expression of H-2K versus H-2D antigens, distinguishing high-metastatic from low-metastatic clones, is correlated with the immunogenic properties of the tumor cells. Int J Cancer 34(4):567–573

Ellis LM, Fidler IJ (2010) Finding the tumor copycat. Therapy fails, patients don't. Nat Med 16(9):974–975

Feldman M, Eisenbach L (1991) MHC class I genes controlling the metastatic phenotype of tumor cells. Semin Cancer Biol 2(5):337–346

Fisher M, Yang LX (2002) Anticancer effects and mechanisms of polysaccharide-K (PSK): implications of cancer immunotherapy. Anticancer Res 22(3):1737–1754

Garrido A, Perez M, Delgado C, Garrido ML, Rojano J, Algarra I, Garrido F (1986a) Influence of class I H-2 gene expression on local tumor growth. Description of a model obtained from clones derived from a solid BALB/c tumor. Exp Clin Immunogenet 3(2):98–110

Garrido ML, Perez M, Delgado C, Rojano J, Algarra I, Garrido A, Garrido F (1986b) Im-munogenicity of H-2 positive and H-2 negative clones of a mouse tumour, GR9. J Immunogenet 13(2–3):159–167

Garrido C, Romero I, Berruguilla E, Cancela B, Algarra I, Collado A, Garcia-Lora A, Garrido F (2011) Immunotherapy eradicates metastases with reversible defects in MHC class I expression. Cancer Immunol Immunother 60(9):1257–1268. doi:10.1007/s00262-011-1027-1

Indrova M, Bieblova J, Jandlova T, Vonka V, Pajtasz-Piasecka E, Reinis M (2006) Chemotherapy, IL-12 gene therapy and combined adjuvant therapy of HPV 16-associated MHC class I-proficient and -deficient tumours. Int J Oncol 28(1):253–259

Indrova M, Simova J, Bieblova J, Bubenik J, Reinis M (2011) NK1.1+ cells are important for the development of protective immunity against MHC I-deficient, HPV16-associated tumours. Oncol Rep 25(1):281–288

Lim YS, Kang BY, Kim EJ, Kim SH, Hwang SY, Kim TS (1998) Augmentation of thera-peutic antitumor immunity by B16F10 melanoma cells transfected by interferon-gamma and alloge-neic MHC class I cDNAs. Mol Cells 8(5):629–636

Lu T, Ramakrishnan R, Altiok S, Youn JI, Cheng P, Celis E, Pisarev V, Sherman S, Sporn MB, Gabrilovich D (2011) Tumor-infiltrating myeloid cells induce tumor cell resistance to cytotoxic T cells in mice. J Clin Invest 121(10):4015–4029

Mandelboim O, Feldman M, Eisenbach L (1992) H-2K double transfectants of tumor cells as antimetastatic cellular vaccines in heterozygous recipients. Implications for the T cell repertoire. J Immunol 148(11):3666–3673

Manning J, Indrova M, Lubyova B, Pribylova H, Bieblova J, Hejnar J, Simova J, Jandlova T, Bubenik J, Reinis M (2008) Induction of MHC class I molecule cell surface expression and epigenetic activation of antigen-processing machinery components in a murine model for human papilloma virus 16-associated tumours. Immunology 123(2):218–227

Perez M, Algarra I, Ljunggren HG, Caballero A, Mialdea MJ, Gaforio JJ, Klein G, Karre K, Garrido F (1990) A weakly tumorigenic phenotype with high MHC class-I expression is associated with high metastatic potential after surgical removal of the primary murine fibrosarcoma. Int J Cancer 46(2):258–261

Plaksin D, Gelber C, Feldman M, Eisenbach L (1988) Reversal of the metastatic phenotype in Lewis lung carcinoma cells after transfection with syngeneic H-2Kb gene. Proc Natl Acad Sci U S A 85(12):4463–4467

Porgador A, Bannerji R, Watanabe Y, Feldman M, Gilboa E, Eisenbach L (1993) Anti-metastatic vaccination of tumor-bearing mice with two types of IFN-gamma gene-inserted tumor cells. J Immunol 150(4):1458–1470

Porgador A, Brenner B, Vadai E, Feldman M, Eisenbach L (1991) Immunization by gamma-IFN-treated B16-F10.9 melanoma cells protects against metastatic spread of the parental tumor. Int J Cancer Suppl 6:54–60

Reinis M, Simova J, Bubenik J (2006) Inhibitory effects of unmethylated CpG oligodeoxynucleotides on MHC class I-deficient and -proficient HPV16-associated tumours. Int J Cancer 118(7):1836–1842

Reinis M, Simova J, Indrova M, Bieblova J, Bubenik J (2007) CpG oligodeoxynucleotides are effective in therapy of minimal residual tumour disease after chemotherapy or surgery in a murine model of MHC class I-deficient, HPV16-associated tumours. Int J Oncol 30(5):1247–1251

Reinis M, Stepanek I, Simova J, Bieblova J, Pribylova H, Indrova M, Bubenik J (2010) Induction of protective immunity against MHC class I-deficient, HPV16-associated tumours with peptide and dendritic cell-based vaccines. Int J Oncol 36(3):545–551

Setiadi AF, Omilusik K, David MD, Seipp RP, Hartikainen J, Gopaul R, Choi KB, Jefferies WA (2008) Epigenetic enhancement of antigen processing and presentation promotes immune recognition of tumors. Cancer Res 68(23):9601–9607

Simova J, Bubenik J, Bieblova J, Rosalia RA, Fric J, Reinis M (2006) Depletion of T(reg) cells inhibits minimal residual disease after surgery of HPV16-associated tumours. Int J Oncol 29(6):1567–1571

Simova J, Pollakova V, Indrova M, Mikyskova R, Bieblova J, Stepanek I, Bubenik J, Reinis M (2011) Immunotherapy augments the effect of 5-azacytidine on HPV16-associated tumours with different MHC class I-expression status. Br J Cancer 105(10):1533–1541. doi:bjc2011428

Sin JI, Park JB, Lee IH, Park D, Choi YS, Choe J, Celis E (2012) Intratumoral electro-poration of IL-12 cDNA eradicates established melanomas by Trp2(180–188)-specific CD8+ CTLs in a perforin/granzyme-mediated and IFN-gamma-dependent manner: application of Trp2(180–188) peptides. Cancer Immunol Immunother 61(10):1671–1682

VandenDriessche T, Bakkus M, Toussaint-Demylle D, Thielemans K, Verschueren H, De Baetselier P (1994a) Tumorigenicity of mouse T lymphoma cells is controlled by the level of major histocompatibility complex class I H-2Kk antigens. Clin Exp Metastasis 12(1):73–83

VandenDriessche T, Geldhof A, Bakkus M, Toussaint-Demylle D, Brijs L, Thielemans K, Verschueren H, De Baetselier P (1994b) Metastasis of mouse T lymphoma cells is controlled by the level of major histocompatibility complex class I H-2Dk antigens. Int J Cancer 58(2):217–225

Chapter 4
Potential Therapeutic Approaches for Increasing Tumor Immunogenicity by Upregulation of Tumor HLA Class I Expression

Based on clinical and experimental evidence it has become clear that low or altered expression of HLA class I molecules on tumor cells are likely to have a negative impact on the outcome of cancer immunotherapy, since it provides malignant cells with a mechanism of immune escape from T cell recognition. Various mechanisms, both reversible and irreversible, underlie the MHC class I down-regulation. Therapies that lead to MHC class I upregulation on tumor cells might improve outcomes in immune-therapy-based treatments. Attempts are in progress to revert the defects in tumor MHC class I surface expression by introducing the elements of the antigen presentation pathway or by activating transcriptional factors that regulate expression of MHC class I molecules or components of APM machinery. It has been demonstrated that IFNs upregulate the expression of MHC class I molecules on cancer cells in vitro and in vivo (Seliger et al. 2000; Martini et al. 2010), unless tumor is resistant to IFN treatment due to genetic defect in IFN signal transduction pathway (Rodriguez et al. 2007). Therefore, IFN treatment is a valuable strategy for cancer immunotherapy aimed at increasing tumor cell immunogenicity, but only in cancer cells that do not harbor structural defects in genes coding for MHC molecules causing loss of class I expression. In that case transfer of a wild type MHC gene into tumor cells is necessary to recover normal MHC-I expression. Epigenetic events associated with tumor development and with cancer progression have been found to underlie changes in HLA antigen and APM components. These alterations can be reversed in vitro with pharmacologic agents that induce DNA hypomethylation or inhibit histone deacetylation (Fonsatti et al. 2007).

In vitro manipulation with $\beta 2m$ gene and with other genes involved in MHC class I complex expression has generated evidence that restoration of normal MHC class I re-expression is important for the tumor cell recognition and elimination by CD8+ T cells. Recovery of MHC class I expression has been employed previously by various investigators to demonstrate the importance of class I molecules in specific tumor lysis by CTL and NK cells. The earliest reports in the 1970s were based on mouse models with known MHC defects. The first description of the loss of an H-2Kk private specificity was reported in Gardener lymphoma derived from a C3H mouse (Garrido et al. 1976). One particular AKR tumor cell line designated K36.16 had no expression of Kk antigen and was resistant to killing by AKR anti-MuLV cytotoxic lymphocytes in vitro, and always produced tumors in immunocompetent AKR mice (Festenstein et al. 1980). In different experimental systems, introduction of MHC class I molecules into MHC class I negative tumor cell lines led to increased immunogenicity of the tumor cells and abrogation of malignancy. The transfection and cell surface expression of an H-2Kk gene in the K36 (H-2Kk negative) lymphoma inhibited the syngeneic growth of this tumor (Hui et al. 1984). Chen and coworkers (1996) analyzed breast and lung cancer for β2m down-regulation or mutations. They identified 63 tumors without detectable β2m mutations and two neoplasms with β2m mutations; they transfected cells with wild type β2m gene and demonstrated complete restoration of HLA expression. They also observed that mutation in β2m caused cell line H2009 to be resistant to specific lysis by influenza virus-specific CTL from HLA matched donors, and that transfection of the β2m gene restored the cytotoxicity. Tafuro and associates (2001) adopted another approach to reconstitute antigen presentation in HLA class I-negative cancer cell lines. They engineered an HLA-A2 restricted peptide epitope linked to the N terminus of β2m and delivered this fusion protein to tumor cells using a retroviral vector. The transfected cells were recognized and killed by appropriate CTL clones. Nabel and colleagues (1996) reported results of a direct transfer of the HLA-B7 gene into HLA-B7-negative patients with advanced melanoma by injection of DNA-liposome complexes (allogeneic vaccination). Plasmid DNA and recombinant HLA-B7 protein were detected in treated tumors. One patient showed a regression of injected nodules after two independent treatments, which was accompanied by regression at distant sites. Bergen and coworkers (2003) reported preliminary results of the clinical trial of HLA-B7/beta-2-microglobulin plasmid DNA/lipid complex (Allovectin-7(R)) in patients with metastatic melanoma. While the clinical outcome of the gene transfer was not dramatic in this case, Allovectin-7 appears to be a promising agent with a safe toxicity profile. However, the main limitation of this type of vaccine is that it is an allogeneic vaccine, not targeted to restoration of a specific gene defect in a given patient. Experiments by Tsory and colleagues (2006) suggested that MHC class I glycoproteins may regulate the immune response by modulating the expression and function of other genes essential for proper antigen processing and presentation. They reported that reconstitution of expression of MHC class I glycoproteins in MHC-deficient and highly metastatic B16BL6 melanoma cells augmented the expression of TAP-2 and inducible proteasome subunits, LMP-2 and LMP-7. Upregulation of inducible proteasome subunits was also followed by a significant change in the proteolytic activity of the proteasome complex. In APM-deficient mouse lung carcinoma cell line CMT.64, re-expression of TAP1 after infection with TAP1-adenovirus vector led to increased MHC class I surface expression, antigen presentation, and susceptibility to antigen-specific CTLs (Lou et al. 2005). Our group designed an adenoviral vector with wild type β2m gene and was able to restore normal HLA class I expression in human tumor cell lines harboring β2m mutations (del Campo et al. 2009). Reconstitution of β2m expression following transduction with the adenovirus was sufficient to restore total HLA class I expression on different human tumor cells lines recovering the lysis of tumor cells by peptide-stimulated HLA-restricted T-cells and increasing peptide-specific IFN-gamma secretion by these T-cells in HLA-restricted manner (del Campo et al. 2012 and unpublished data).

Epigenetic events associated with tumor development and with cancer progression have been also found to underlie changes in HLA antigen and APM components. DNA methylation was found to be responsible for the MHC class I heavy chain gene inhibition (Nie et al. 2001; Serrano et al. 2001), while both the DNA methylation and histone acetylation changes were associated with inhibition of the antigen presenting machinery (APM) gene expression (Campoli and Ferrone 2008).These alterations can be reversed in vitro with pharmacologic agents that induce DNA hypomethylation or inhibit histone deacetylation (Fonsatti et al. 2007). The therapeutic benefit of such "epigenetic" agents, including histone deacetylase and DNA methyltransferase inhibitors (DNMTi), has been successfully tested in clinical trials and several compounds, including DNMTi 5-azacytidine (5AC) and 5-aza-2-deoxycytidine (DAC) have been approved for clinical use (Mai and Altucci 2009).

There is an accumulating body of evidence suggesting that a combination of different types of cancer therapy, including chemotherapy, immunotherapy and gene therapy aimed at recovering normal HLA class I expression, gives the best results in both animal models and in clinical trials. Such a combined therapy may have some advantages in combating well-established tumors and metastatic cancer.

References

Bergen M, Chen R, Gonzalez R (2003) Efficacy and safety of HLA-B7/beta-2 microglobulin plasmid DNA/lipid complex (Allovectin-7) in patients with metastatic melanoma. Expert Opin Biol Ther 3(2):377–384

Campoli M, Ferrone S (2008) HLA antigen changes in malignant cells: epigenetic mechanisms and biologic significance. Oncogene 27(45):5869–5885

Chen HL, Gabrilovich D, Virmani A, Ratnani I, Girgis KR, Nadaf-Rahrov S, Fernandez-Viña M, Carbone DP (1996) Structural and functional analysis of beta2 microglobulin abnormalities in human lung and breast cancer. Int J Cancer 67(6):756 763

del Campo AB, Aptsiauri N, Méndez R, Zinchenko S, Vales A, Paschen A, Ward S, Ruiz-Cabello F, González-Aseguinolaza G, Garrido F (2009) Efficient recovery of HLA class I expression in human tumor cells after beta2-microglobulin gene transfer using adenoviral vector: implications for cancer immunotherapy. Scand J Immunol 70(2):125–135

del Campo AB, Carretero J, Aptsiauri N, Garrido F (2012) Targeting HLA class I expression to increase tumor immunogenicity. Tissue Antigens 79(3):147–154

Festenstein H, Schmidt W, Testorelli C, Marelli O, Simpson S (1980) Biologic effects of the altered MHS profile on the K36 tumor, a spontaneous leukemia of AKR. Transplant Proc 12(1):25 28

Fonsatti E, Nicolay HJ, Sigalotti L, Calabrò L, Pezzani L, Colizzi F, Altomonte M, Guidoboni M, Marincola FM, Maio M (2007) Functional up-regulation of human leukocyte antigen class I antigens expression by 5-aza-2'-deoxycytidine in cutaneous melanoma: immunotherapeutic implications. Clin Cancer Res 13(11):3333–3338

Garrido F, Festenstein H, Schirrmacher V (1976) Further evidence for depression of H-2 and Ia-like specificities of foreign haplotypes in mouse tumour cell lines. Nature 261(5562):705–707

Hui K, Grosveld F, Festenstein H (1984) Rejection of transplantable AKR leukaemia cells following MHC DNA-mediated cell transformation. Nature 311(5988):750–752

Lou Y, Vitalis TZ, Basha G, Cai B, Chen SS, Choi KB, Jeffries AP, Elliott WM, Atkins D, Seliger B, Jefferies WA (2005) Restoration of the expression of transporters associated with antigen processing in lung carcinoma increases tumor-specific immune responses and survival. Cancer Res 65(17):7926–7933

Mai A, Altucci L (2009) Epi-drugs to fight cancer: from chemistry to cancer treatment, the road ahead. Int J Biochem Cell Biol 41:199–213

Martini M, Testi MG, Pasetto M, Picchio MC, Innamorati G, Mazzocco M, Ugel S, Cingarlini S, Bronte V, Zanovello P, Krampera M, Mosna F, Cestari T, Riviera AP, Brutti N, Barbieri O, Matera L, Tridente G, Colombatti M, Sartoris S (2010) IFN-gamma-mediated upmodulation of MHC class I expression activates tumor-specific immune response in a mouse model of prostate cancer. Vaccine 28:3548–3557

Nabel GJ, Gordon D, Bishop DK, Nickoloff BJ, Yang ZY, Aruga A, Cameron MJ, Nabel EG, Chang AE (1996) Immune response in human melanoma after transfer of an allogeneic class I major histocompatibility complex gene with DNA-liposome complexes. Proc Natl Acad Sci U S A 93(26):15388–15393

Nie Y, Yang G, Song Y, Zhao X, So C, Liao J, Wang LD, Yang CS (2001) DNA hypermethylation is a mechanism for loss of expression of the HLA class I genes in human esophageal squamous cell carcinomas. Carcinogenesis 22(10):1615–1623

Rodriguez T, Mendez R, Del Campo A, Jimenez P, Aptsiauri N, Garrido F, Ruiz-Cabello F (2007) Distinct mechanisms of loss of IFN-gamma mediated HLA class I inducibility in two melanoma cell lines. BMC Cancer 7:34

Seliger B, Maeurer MJ, Ferrone S (2000) Antigen-processing machinery breakdown and tumor growth. Immunol Today 21(9):455–464

Serrano A, Tanzarella S, Lionello I, Mendez R, Traversari C, Ruiz-Cabello F, Garrido F (2001) Rexpression of HLA class I antigens and restoration of antigen-specific CTL response in melanoma cells following 5-aza-2′-deoxycytidine treatment. Int J Cancer 94(2):243–251

Tafuro S, Meier UC, Dunbar PR, Jones EY, Layton GT, Hunter MG, Bell JI, McMichael AJ (2001) Reconstitution of antigen presentation in HLA class I-negative cancer cells with peptide-beta2m fusion molecules. Eur J Immunol 31(2):440–449

Tsory S, Kellman-Pressman S, Fishman D, Segal S (2006) Reconstitution of expression of H-2K region-encoded murine MHC class I glycoproteins in MHC class I-deficient B16BL6 melanoma cells affects the expression and function of antigen-processing machinery. Immunol Lett 102(2):237–240

Chapter 5
Conclusions

Altered MHC Class I expression is a hallmark of malignant transformation and tumor immune escape. Using immunohistochemistry and molecular techniques it has been demonstrated that many types of tumor can lose up to 80 % of normal MHC class I expression. Both reversible and irreversible structural defects of MHC class I have been described in solid tumors, in cancer cell lines and metastatic lesions. As a result, malignant cells develop low immunogenic phenotypes with altered antigen-presentation ability. It leads to the loss of tumor recognition by cytotoxic T lymphocytes, providing an immune escape route for MHC-negative cells, and limits the efficacy of cancer immunotherapy. A growing body of evidence supports a hypothesis that the irreversible genetic defects underlying abnormal MHC expression are, at least partially, responsible for the emergence of immunotherapy-resistant tumor escape variants. We have obtained clinical data demonstrating that progressing melanoma metastases that develop after immuno-therapy have more alterations causing abnormal HLA class I expression that lesions that regress. Similarly, recurrent bladder tumors developed after BCG therapy showed more profound genetic defects in HLA class I molecules. Results obtained from cancer animal models also support the importance of MHC class I expression in response to therapy. These results indicate that the success of immunotherapy as anti-metastatic treatment may depend strongly of the MHC I expression level on primary tumor cells. Thus, in our era of "personalized medicine" it seems to be important to include tumor MHC expression into the list of biomarkers to be closely monitored before, during and after cancer immunotherapy to increase the clinical efficacy of the treatment. It is also important to develop more uniform techniques of the tumor MHC class I expression and more consistent ways to interpret the data. We believe that a combination of immunotherapy with chemotherapy and gene therapy is the most promising approach in fighting cancer.

N. Aptsiauri et al., *MHC Class I Antigens In Malignant Cells: Immune Escape and Response to Immunotherapy*, SpringerBriefs in Cancer Research 6, DOI 10.1007/978-1-4614-6543-0_5, © Teresa Cabrera 2013